Podiatric Medicine and Surgery
A Monograph series

Edited by

Morton D. Fielding, D.P.M.

Volume I : The Surgical Treatment of the Hallux-Abducto Valgus
Volume II: The Surgical Treatment of the Intractable Plantar Keratoma

The Surgical Treatment of the Intractable Plantar Keratoma

Edited by

Morton D. Fielding, D.P.M.
Consulting Podiatrist to the National Institute of Health

Contributors

Joshua Gerbert, D.P.M., M.S.
Thomas Melillo, D.P.M., M.S.
Tilden Sokoloff, D.P.M., M.S.
Eugene Spector, D.P.M., M.S.
Alan K. Whitney, D.P.M.

FUTURA
PUBLISHING COMPANY
1974

Published by
Futura Publishing Company, Inc.
295 Main Street
Mount Kisco, New York 10549

L.C.: 74-79948
ISBN: 0-87993-040-3

This volume is dedicated to the 1974 senior classes of all the colleges of Podiatric Medicine in the United States.

It is to their future that we dedicate this book.

Contributors

Donald K. Alexander, D.P.M.

Joshua Gerbert, D.P.M., M.S.
Associate Professor; Director, Department of Podiatric Surgery; Director of Second Year Surgical Residency Program; California College of Podiatric Medicine, San Francisco

Thomas Melillo, D.P.M., M.S.
Co-chief and Associate Professor, Department of Surgery and Biomechanics, Pennsylvania College of Podiatric Medicine

Tilden Sokoloff, D.P.M., M.S.
Professor, Department of Podiatric Surgery; Professor, Department of Podiatric Biomechanics; Immediate Past Chairman, Department of Podiatric Surgery, California College of Podiatric Medicine, San Francisco

Eugene Spector, D.P.M., M.S.
Associate Professor of Surgery; Assistant Director, Department of Surgery, California College of Podiatric Medicine

Alan K. Whitney, D.P.M.
Director, Division of Allied Health Programs; Director, Podiatric Assistants Program; Professor of Podiatry; Surgical Staff Pennsylvania College of Podiatric Medicine

Preface

In this, our second monograph, "The Surgical Treatment of the Intractable Plantar Keratoma", we have attempted to cover in surgical detail one of the most common foot ailments seen in our offices. There are twenty-seven surgical procedures for the surgeon to choose from, depending upon the location of the keratoma and the biomechanical considerations necessary.

In order to use this monograph as a quick perusal reference, the book is sectioned in such a manner as to quickly facilitate the choice of procedure for the keratoma to be removed.

In the book you will notice the interchangeable usage of the words keratoma or keratoses. After spending hours in researching these words with the able assistance of David M. Goff, D.P.M., it is the conclusion of the editor that the terms are synonymous and can be used interchangeably. Keratoma is a newer terminology and seems to have wider usage in podiatry, particularly in the mid and far western regions of the United States. Keratoses is the older term and is most frequently found used in dermatology and in the eastern podiatric regions.

Section I consists of a close up anatomy of the forefoot very ably drawn and illustrated by Dr. Alan K. Whitney.

Section II deals with the biomechanical consideration, including radiographic examination and evaluation.

Dr. Tilden Sokoloff wrote the biomechanical section with drawings by Dr. S. Newell.

Dr. Joshua Gerbert wrote the radiographic examination and evaluation.

Section III has been divided into three separate areas.

Part A, Surgical Procedures for First Metatarsal IPK, lists six procedures:

Dr. Joshua Gerbert wrote the procedures for tibial and fibular sesamoidectomy.

Dr. Eugene Spector wrote the procedures on dorsal wedge osteotomy, biplace osteotomy and Sir Robert Jones procedure.

Dr. Thomas Melillo wrote the procedure on crescentic osteotomy.

Part B, Second, Third and Fourth Metatarsal IPK, has eight procedures listed:

Dr. Joshua Gerbert wrote the procedures for extension osteoarthrotomy (EOA).

Dr. Eugene Spector wrote the procedures for step down or shortening osteotomy, V-Osteotomy at neck of metatarsal and the plantar condylectomy.

Dr. Thomas Melillo wrote the procedures for crescentic osteotomy of the lesser metatarsals and the metatarsal head resection.

Dr. Tilden Sokoloff wrote the procedure on dorsal wedge osteotomy of the lesser metatarsals.

Dr. Donald Alexander wrote the procedure on open metaphyseal osteotomy.

Part C, Fifth Metatarsal IPK, has seven procedures listed:

Dr. Joshua Gerbert wrote the procedure on adductory wedge osteotomy, dorsal wedge osteotomy and biplane osteotomy.

Dr. Thomas Melillo wrote the procedures on plantar condylectomy, lateral condylectomy, and fifth metatarsal head resection.

Dr. Donald Alexander wrote the procedures on open metaphyseal osteotomy.

Part D, Pan Metatarsal Head Resection for IPK, was written by Dr. Joshua Gerbert.

Section IV, Soft Tissue Procedures, was written by Dr. Alan K. Whitney.

Section V, Procedures Less Commonly Performed, has three different procedures written and critiqued.

Dr. Joshua Gerbert wrote on the peg and hole procedure.

Dr. Alan K. Whitney wrote on the collectomy procedure.

Dr. Thomas Melillo wrote on the floating of the metatarsals procedure.

Throughout this monograph the drawings have been done by Drs. Joshua Gerbert and Alan Whitney.

I wish to extend my sincere gratitude, not only to those distinguished colleagues who have prepared the chapters for this book, but also to a number of medical secretaries in their offices who have given generously of their time in typing and retyping the manuscripts. I especially wish to acknowledge my secretary, Mrs. Marcene Michaelson who found the elusive twenty five hour day.

In the preparation of this book, no expression of gratitude would be complete without a special thanks to our lovely wives who have stood by and made many personal sacrifices to allow us to pursue our professional endeavors. Thank you, Phyllis, Francine, Barbara, Judy, Sparky, and Loretta.

MORTON D. FIELDING, D.P.M.

CONTENTS

SECTION I

SURGICAL ANATOMY OF THE FOREFOOT

Surgical Anatomy of the Forefoot

The majority of surgical procedures on the forefoot are performed through a dorsal approach to avoid scars on the plantar surface. Incisions placed over the metatarsophalangeal joints must cross the superficial dorsal venous network, inviting the wound disrupting consequences of ecchymosis and hematoma. Additionally, the dorsal cutaneous nerves must be protected if post-operative paresthesia or neuralgia is to be avoided. A detailed knowledge of human forefoot anatomy and the common variations encountered should be the possession of every surgeon entering this complex region.

Herein is a series of illustrations depicting the various tissues and structures to be found at increasing depths in the forefoot, as visualized through the dorsal approach. It is hoped that this visual presentation of forefoot anatomy will serve the need for review of a selected area of surgical intervention.

The skin of the dorsum is relatively thin, attaining 2- to 3-mm thickness, and normally possesses good kinetic rebound or turgor. The ectomorph displays a more delicate integument than the endomorph. Numerous cutaneous nerve endings for pain, touch, and temperature exist on the dorsum but are more sparse than on the plantar surface. Hair distribution is normally limited to the medial dorsum and over the proximal phalanges in hirsuitous individuals. DuVries indicates the pattern of normal *skin cleavage lines* to be more or less longitudinal and curvilinear from the first segment. Dorsal incisions are best made along skin cleavage lines, and longitudinal in direction so as to avoid injury to cutaneous nerves.

The plantar skin is profusely laden with exteroceptive and proprioceptive sensors. It is a unique sensory organ which, reputedly, resists implantation of epidermis from other body areas. Plantar skin is typically thick, approaching 5 to 6 mm. at the ball and heel areas in some individuals. Dynamic weightbearing pressures and tensions tend to disrupt plantar incisions which may then develop prominent and painful scars.

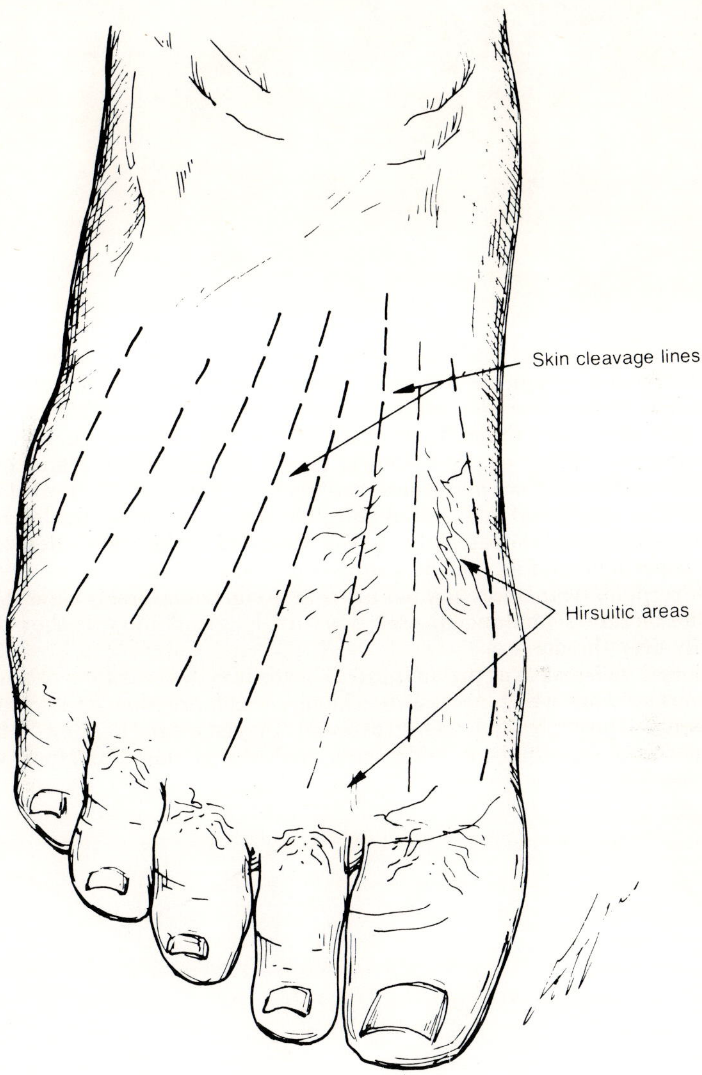

FIGURE 1
EPIDERMIS

The medial and lateral *dorsal digital veins* drain, proximally, into a highly variable and irregular network of superficial veins — the *dorsal venous network*. Interconnections show numerous arching and forking patterns that are only visualized, topically, through the most delicate integuments. From the proximal boundary of the network, larger arcuate veins drain toward both medial and lateral foot margins as the *marginal foot veins*. In front of the medial malleolus, the dorsal and medial marginal tributaries enter the leg as the *great saphenous vein* while, laterally, they pass behind the lateral malleolus to ascend the superficial calf as the *short saphenous vein*.

Superficial lymphatic channels are said to run transversely across the dorsum of the metatarsophalangeal area but turn longitudinally as they pass proximally over the dorsum.

Dorsal incisions over the metatarsal heads inevitably transect the superficial venous network which necessitates hemostat compression, or at times ligation, to forestall postoperative ecchymosis and delayed wound healing. Total forefoot hemostasis, from incision to dressing, makes such vascular repair difficult to impossible.

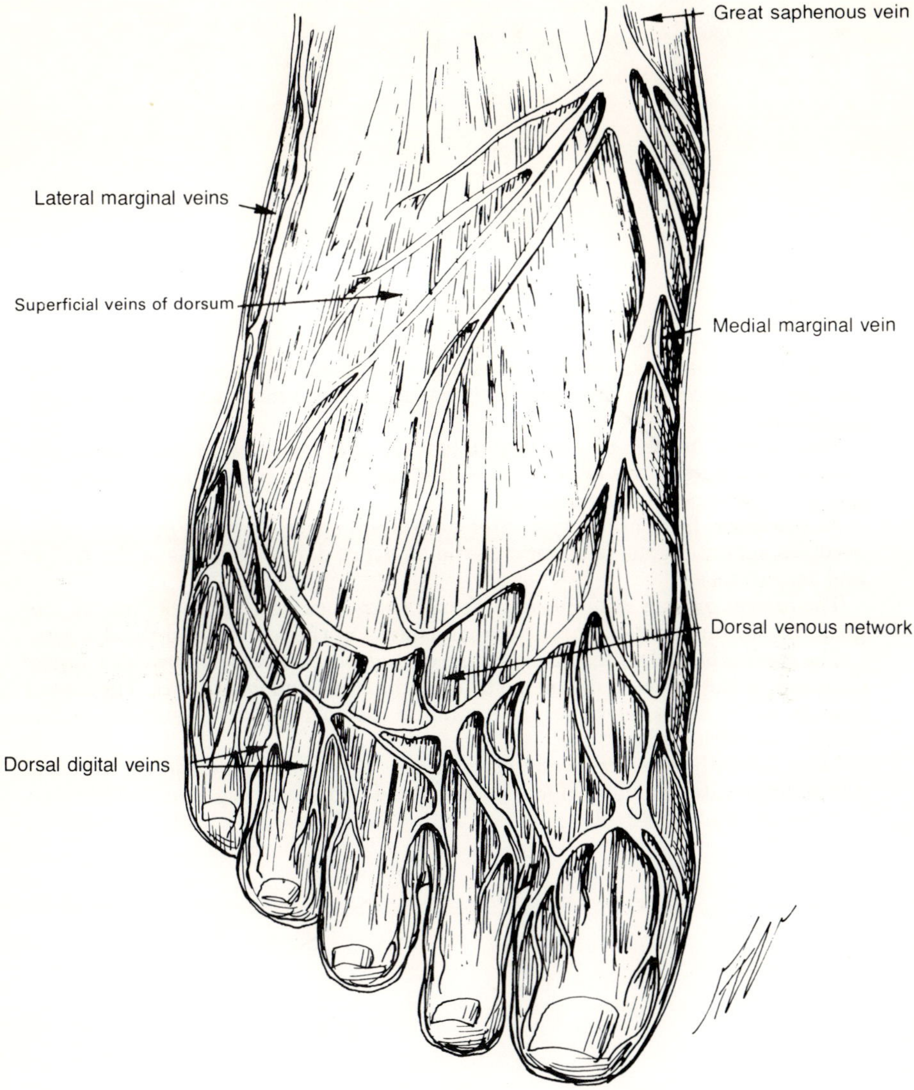

FIGURE 2
SUPERFICIAL DORSAL VENOUS NETWORK

The cutaneous nerves of the dorsum are superficial but deep to the majority of the superficial veins. They are fairly constant rectilinear, and generally longitudinal.

The *medial branch of the medial dorsal cutaneous nerve* runs obliquely medialward across the shaft of the first metatarsal to terminate along the dorsomedial aspect of the hallux.

At the distal level of the first intermetatarsal space, the *deep peroneal nerve* becomes subcutaneous to innervate the adjacent dorsal surfaces of the hallux and second toes.

The *lateral branch of the medial dorsal cutaneous nerve* passes directly longitudinal to innervate adjacent dorsal aspects of the second and third digits.

The *medial branch of the intermediate dorsal cutaneous nerve* provides digital divisions to the adjacent dorsal surfaces of the third and fourth toes. The *lateral branch* of the same nerve serves similarly the corresponding surfaces of the fourth and fifth digits.

More laterally, the *lateral dorsal cutaneous nerve,* a continuation of the sural nerve, innervates the lateral foot border and dorsolateral aspect of the fifth toe.

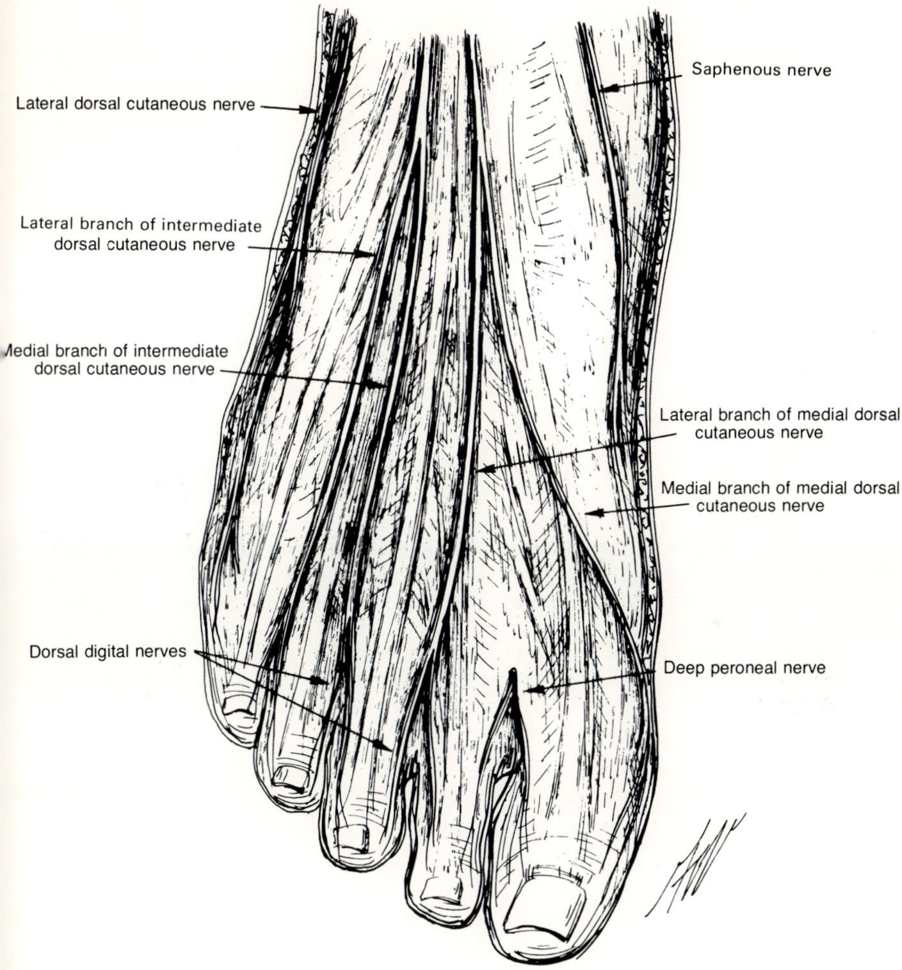

FIGURE 3
DORSAL AND MARGINAL CUTANEOUS NERVES

The long extensor tendons to the hallux and to the four lesser toes possess a *synovial sheath* which usually terminates short of the metatarsophalangeal joint level. As the tendons approach that joint level, they become bound to the articulation by a demonstrable tent-like sheath of fibrous tissue — the *extensor hood ligament* which invests the joint and attaches, plantarly, to the glenoid ligament.

At the midshaft level of the proximal phalanx, the long extensor tendons of the second, third, and fourth toes receive the insertion from tendons of the extensor digitorum brevis muscle. At the hallux, however, the first brevis tendon commonly inserts into the shaft of the proximal phalanx itself. Dorsally, the *long extensor tendons* become intimately blended with the interphalangeal capsules enroute to their final insertion into the dorsal aspect of the distal phalanges.

Functionally, the extensor digitorum longus muscle is a fair extensor of the toes but is considered relatively impotent in its action upon the interphalangeal articulations.

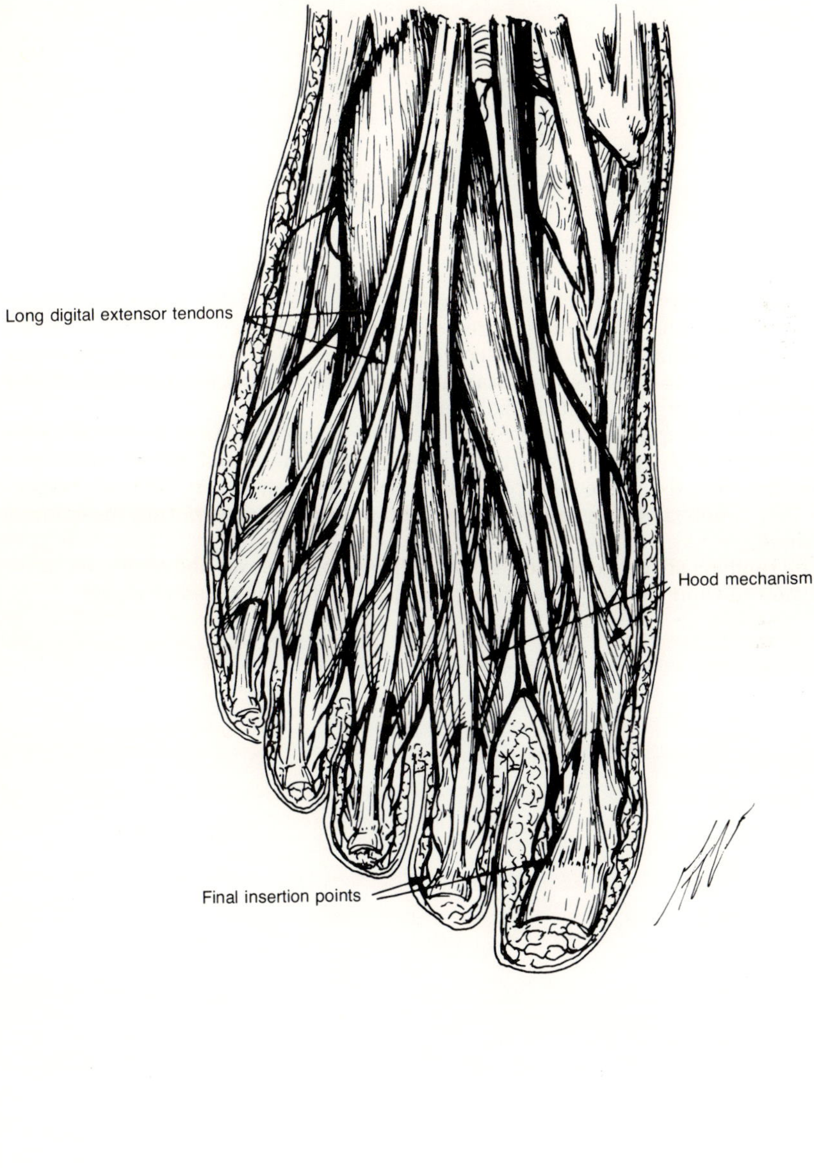

FIGURE 4
LONG DIGITAL EXTENSOR TENDONS AND HOOD MECHANISM

As the exclusive dorsal intrinsic muscle, the *extensor digitorum brevis* presents four tendons which act on the hallux and the three intermediate digits.

The most medial tendon slip, termed the *extensor hallucis brevis,* runs somewhat deeply into the first metatarsal interspace toward its insertion on the proximal phalangeal shaft, dorsolaterally.

The remaining *three lateral brevis tendons* also run rather deeply to their insertions into the corresponding long tendons of the second, third, and fourth toes. Occasionally, these lesser brevis tendons are seen to parallel their respective long tendons all the way to the distal phalanges where mutual insertion is attained.

The tendons of the extensor digitorum brevis produce an abductory vector in addition to their primary dorsiflexion action on the four medial digits.

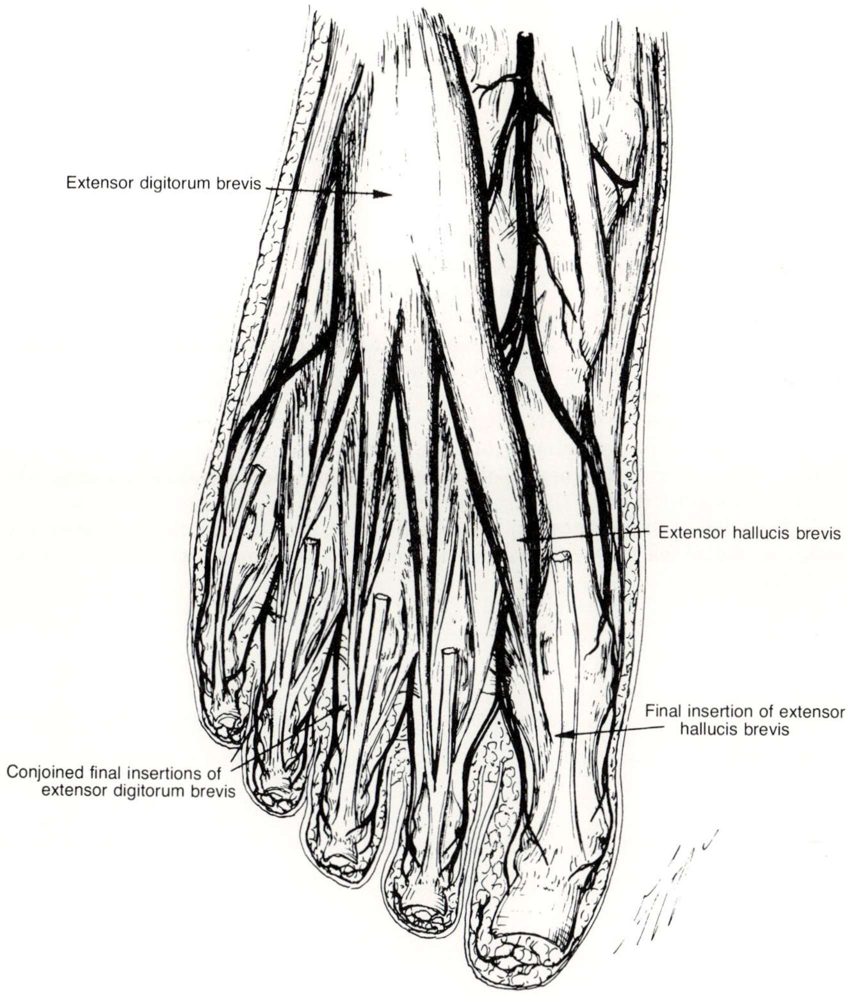

FIGURE 5
EXTENSOR DIGITORUM BREVIS

The *dorsalis pedis artery,* at tarsometatarsal level, curves lateralward as the arcuate artery and gives off four *deep plantar perforating arteries* at the proximal metatarsal interspaces. Four *dorsal metatarsal arteries,* also given off from the arcuate, pass forward beneath and between the interosseous muscles of each interspace to terminate by division into the digital branches supplying adjacent toes. The *dorsal digital arteries* join their plantar counterparts in a glomus union at the toe bulb.

The medial aspect of the first segment and dorsomedial surface of the hallux is usually supplied by an artery from the dorsalis pedis or the dorsalis hallucis artery. The lateral side of the fifth segment and dorsolateral aspect of the quintus is supplied from the arcuate or the fourth dorsal metatarsal artery.

At the level of the metatarsophalangeal joints, each dorsal metatarsal artery sends a *distal plantar perforating artery* to anastomose with the plantar metatarsal vessels.

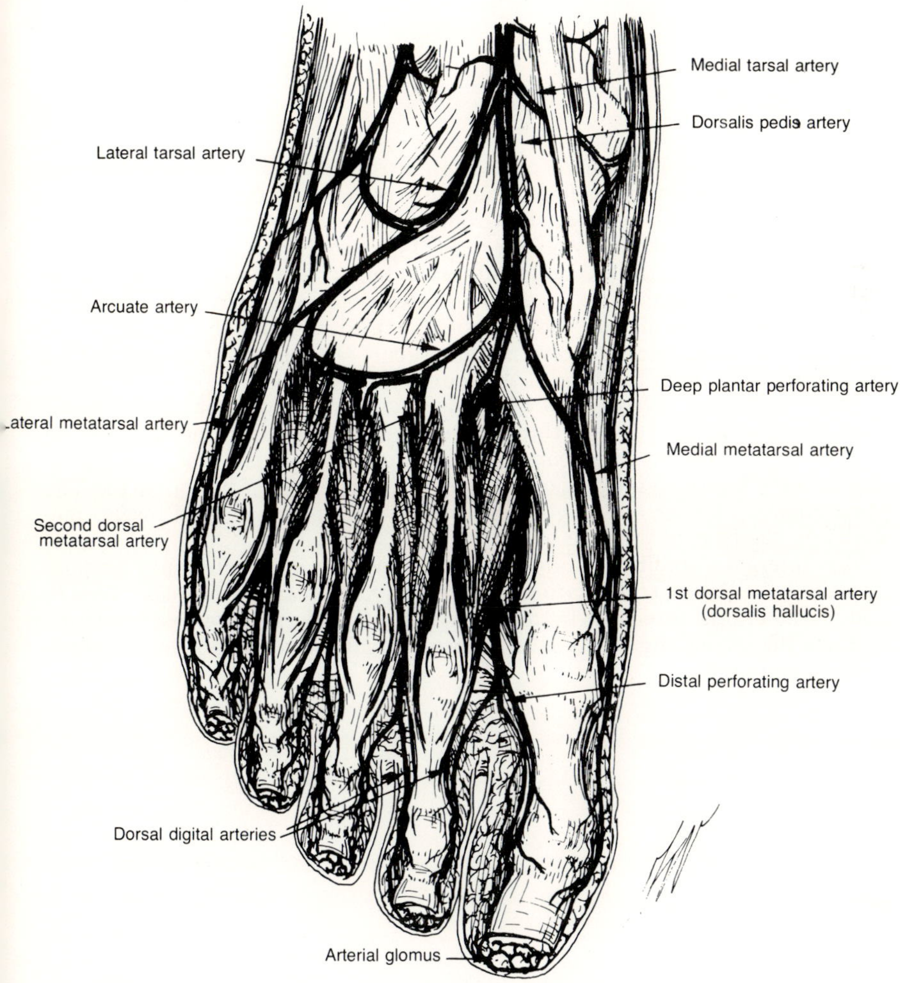

FIGURE 6
DORSAL ARTERIES

There are three unipennate plantar interossei and four bipennate dorsal interosseous muscles in the fourth muscle layer of the sole.

The *first dorsal interosseous* arises from adjacent metatarsal bones in the first interspace to insert medially on the base of the second toe. The *second dorsal interosseous* arises in the second metatarsal interspace to insert laterally on the base of the second digit. The *third dorsal interosseous* arises in the third interspace to insert laterally on the base of the third toe, and the *fourth dorsal interosseous* stems from adjacent metatarsals of the fourth interspace to find insertion laterally on the base of the fourth toe.

The *first plantar interosseous* arises deep to the second dorsal interosseous from the medial aspect of the third metatarsal shaft to insert medially on the base of the third digit. The *second plantar interosseous* arises from the medial aspect of the fourth metatarsal to insert on the medial base of the fourth toe. The *third plantar interosseous* originates in the fourth interspace and inserts medially on the base of the fifth toe.

The interossei exhibit a mild flexory component but their main purpose appears to be that of stabilization. Additionally, the plantar interossei tend to adduct the lateral three toes in concert with the first dorsal interosseous which adducts the second digit. The lateral three dorsal interossei abduct the three intermediate toes.

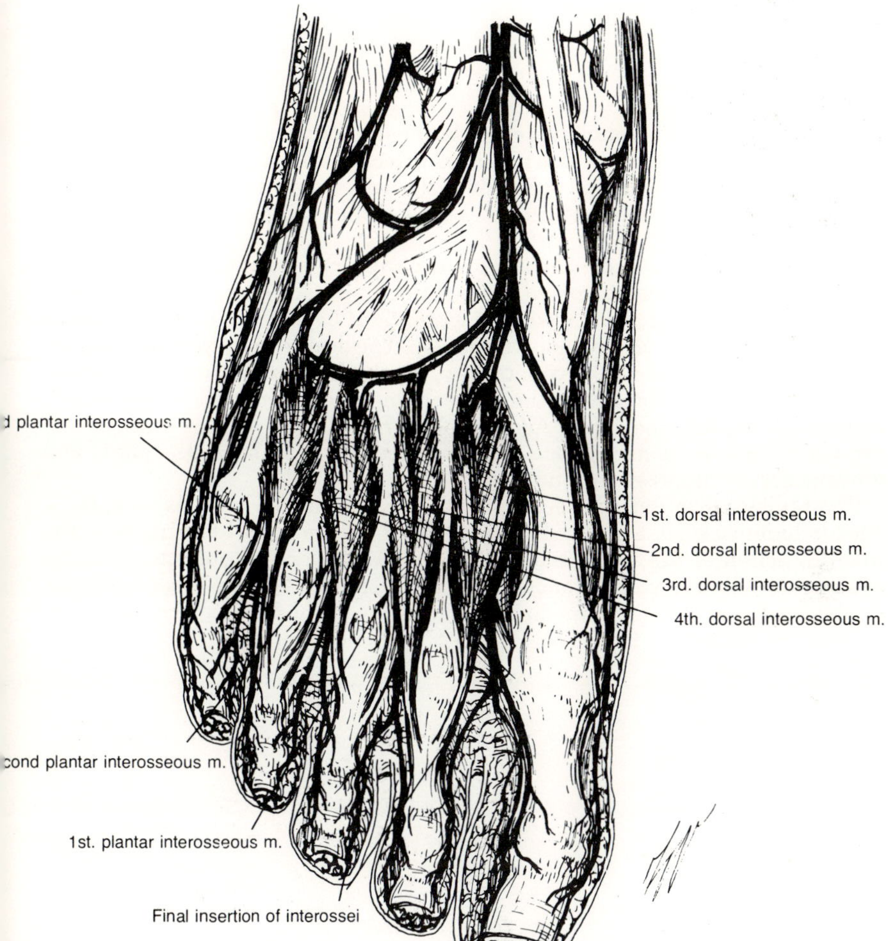

FIGURE 7
INTEROSSEOUS MUSCLES

The normal metatarsophalangeal relationship is one of mild dorsiflexion, corresponding in degree with the metatarsal declination angles. In a transverse plane, the hallux and second toe abduct slightly, the third digit is relatively collinear, while the fourth and fifth toes show adduction from their corresponding metatarsal axis.

The *metatarsophalangeal articulations* are supported dorsally by the *capsules* and the tenofibrous *hood ligaments* descending from each long extensor tendon. The sides of the joints are braced by the *collateral ligaments* and by the dorsal hood expansions which envelop the joints. The lesser metatarsophalangeal joints are further stabilized, collaterally, by the interosseous muscles. Plantarly, the joints are secured by the fibrocartilaginous *glenoid ligaments* which extend distally into the digits. Additionally, the intrinsic plantar muscles and extrinsic flexor tendons produce a balance serving to stabilize the joints and prevent dorsal subluxation tendency.

Plantar stabilization of the first metatarsophalangeal joint is unique. A "flexor hammock" is enhanced by the *radial sesamoids* which improve the fulcrum action of the flexor hallucis brevis. Medially, the abductor hallucis opposes an abductory drift tendency while, laterally, the conjoined adductor hallucis complex prohibits medial displacement of the hallus. The joints are secured, transversely, by the *transverse metatarsal ligaments.*

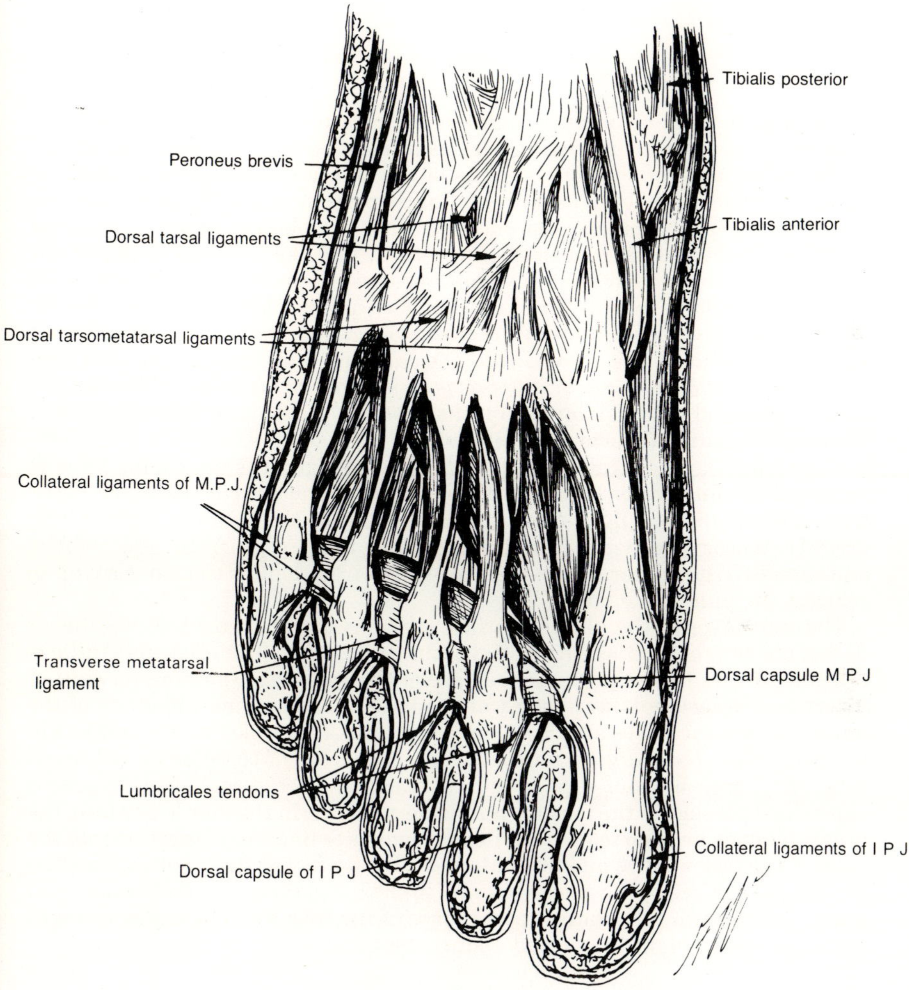

FIGURE 8
METATARSO-PHALANGEAL JOINTS

The fourth layer of intrinsic plantar musculature has been described and illustrated at a more superficial level as considered from a dorsal approach.

The third layer of the sole consists of the flexor hallucis brevis, adductor hallucis complex, and the flexor digiti quinti brevis muscles. The *flexor hallucis brevis* arises from a broad area encompassing the plantar aspect of the first segment. It presents a dual head of insertion into the basal tubercles of the proximal phalanx; each head division encloses a sesamoid which serves for weightbearing and increases the efficiency of hallux plantar flexion. The oblique and transverse portions of the *adductor hallucis* combine to insert, with the lateral head of the brevis, into the lateroplantar base of the proximal phalanx. The *flexor digiti quinti brevis* arises near the bases of the lateral metatarsals and inserts laterally on the base of the fifth proximal phalanx. It plantar flexes and abducts the quintus.

The second layer includes the *four lumbricales* and the *quadratus plantae* muscle. The lumbricales arise from the long flexor tendons, pass plantarly of the transverse metatarsal ligaments to insert dorsally on the expansions of the long digital extensor tendons. The quadratus plantae takes origin from the calcaneus and inserts posterolaterally on the flexor digitorum longus tendon, serving to redirect the pull of the latter.

The first layer of the planter surface contains the abductor hallucis, flexor digitorum brevis, and abductor digiti quinti muscles. The *abductor hallucis* takes its origin from the medial surface of the calcaneus, passing forward to insert on the medioplantar aspect of the base of the proximal phalanx of the hallux. It plantar flexes and "adducts" the hallux in relation to the mid-line of the body. The *flexor digitorum brevis* arises in front of the plantar calcaneal tuberosity, presents four slips that divide near the metatarsal heads to permit superficial passage of the long digital flexor tendons. In the four lesser toes, the brevis tendons lie deep to the long flexor tendons to find their insertion into the sides of the bases of the middle phalanges. The *abductor digiti quinti* arises on the lateral surface of the calcaneus and inserts, together with the flexor digiti quinti brevis, into the plantar lateral base of the fifth toe. The abductor digiti quinti serves to plantar flex and abduct the quintus.

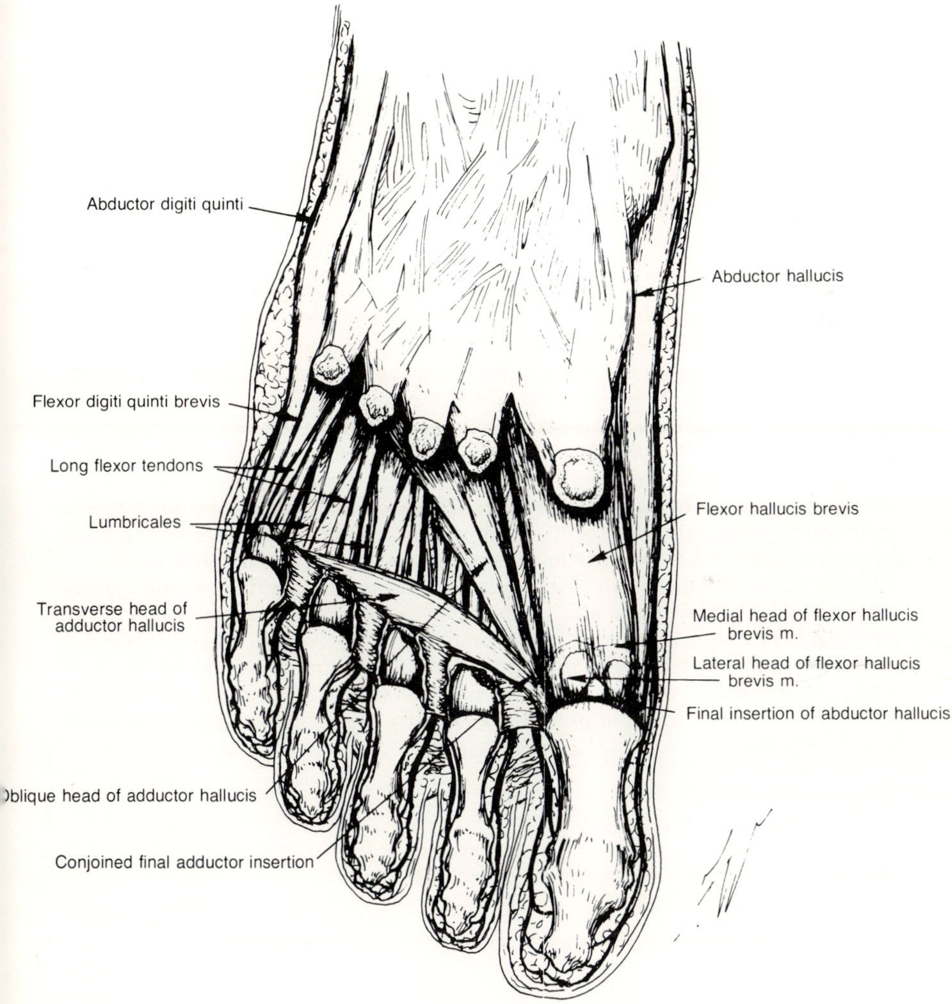

FIGURE 9
PLANTAR INTRINSIC MUSCLES

Of interest to the foot surgeon are the various osseous landmarks and references for sites of prospective osteotomy, ostectomy, and arthroplasty.

The *surgical neck* of the metatarsal exists at a level just distal of the dorsal tubercles of the head and is the site for conservative head resection, or "short capitectomy." The *anatomic neck* is the narrowest portion of the distal shaft, the anterior limit of which is the level for total resection of the metatarsal head, or "long capitectomy." The *free base* of the metatarsals is at a level where the base shows no contact with adjacent metatarsals and is the usual site for angulation or crescentic osteotomies. Tarsometatarsal arthroplasty and arthrectomy levels are found approximately one centimeter proximal of the free base level except at the second segment where the base is elongated and markedly recessed.

The location and direction of individual metatarsals and their related joints can, at times, be deceptive and misleading to the unwary surgeon who may misplace his incision and access to the proposed operative site. Careful, manual palpation of the metatarsal shafts and the neighboring joints forestalls such surgical indiscretion and facilitates precise placement of incisions for the optimal approach to the selected procedure. Equally cautious roentgen correlation is well advised.

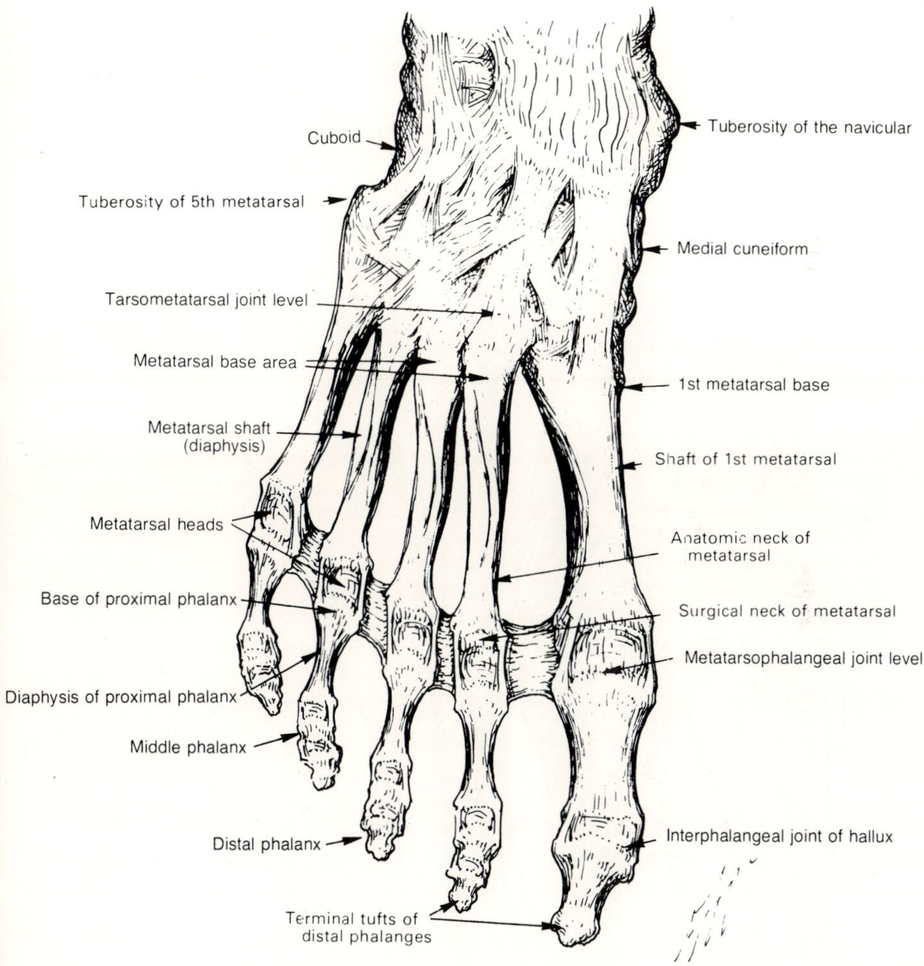

FIGURE 10
FOOT SKELETON

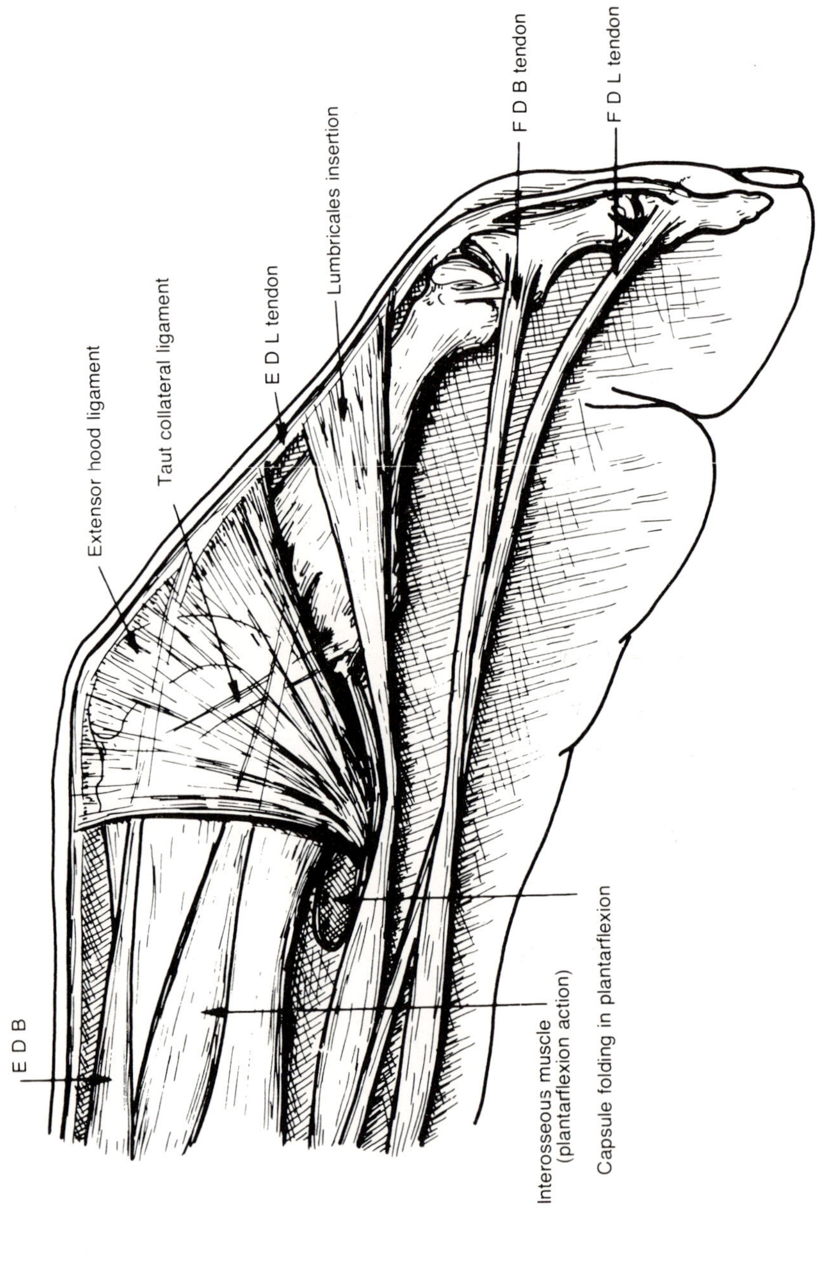

FIGURE 11
CLOSE-UP ANATOMY OF THE METATARSO-PHALANGEAL JOINT IN PLANTARFLEXION

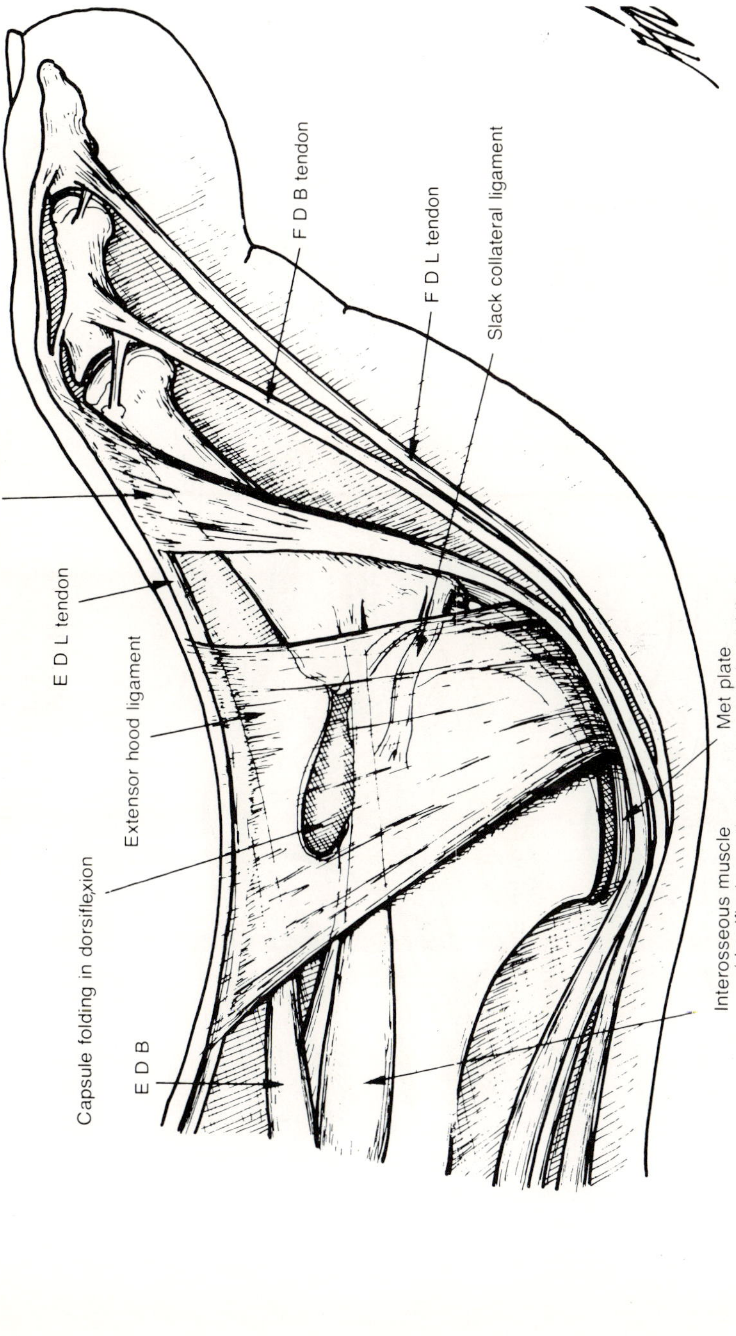

FIGURE 12
CLOSE-UP ANATOMY OF THE METATARSO-PHALANGEAL JOINT IN DORSIFLEXION

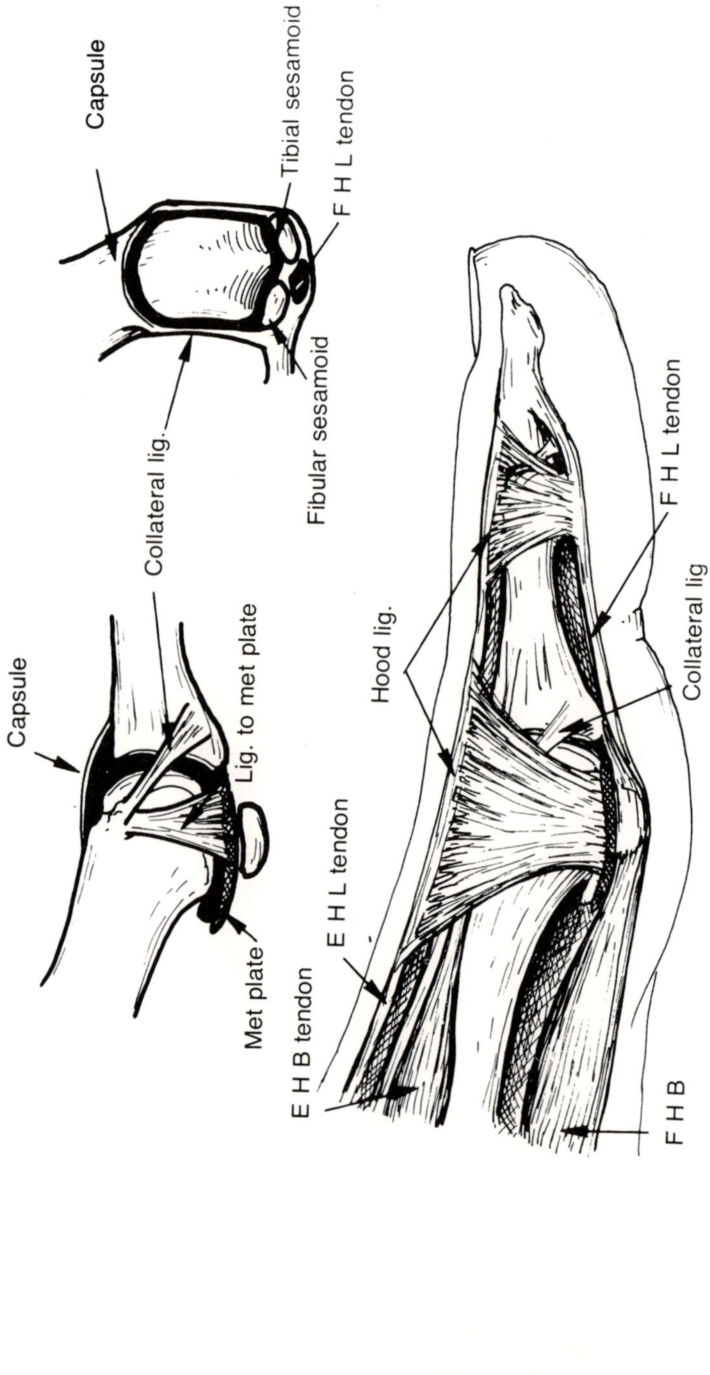

FIGURE 13
CLOSE-UP ANATOMY OF THE
1st METATARSO-PHALANGEAL JOINT

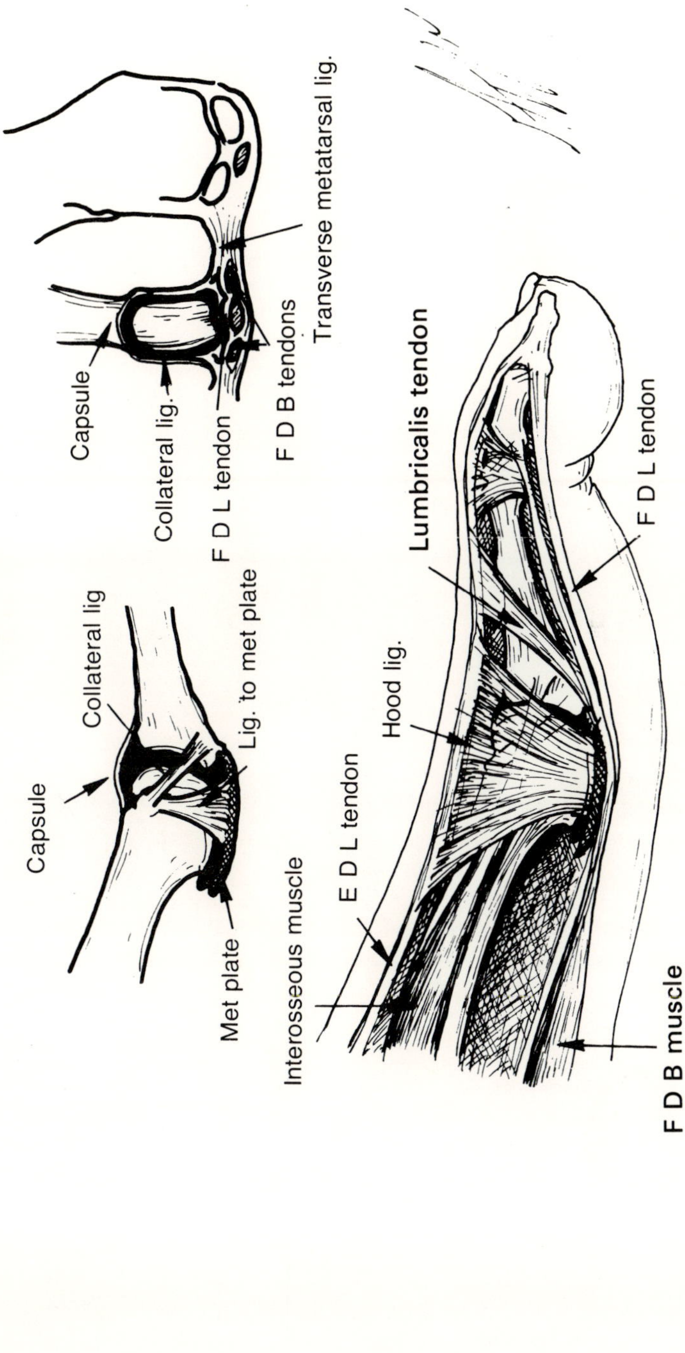

FIGURE 14
CLOSE-UP ANATOMY OF THE LESSER METATARSO-PHALANGEAL JOINTS

SECTION II

BIOMECHANICAL CONSIDERATIONS

RADIOGRAPHIC EXAMINATION AND EVALUATION

A. Biomechanical Considerations

Introduction

The topic of intractable plantar keratosis can not be approached from a surgical view point or a mechanical view point, unless the physician understands the biomechanics of the entire lower extremity. It is incumbent upon the surgeon to understand the etiology of the intractable plantar lesion being approached, not just from a cause and effect, but from structure and function attitude. An intractable plantar keratoma is usually defined as a large hyperkeratotic lesion which is a hypertrophy of the stratum corneum. The lesions usually become painful due to an adventitious bursal sac, which lies plantar to the lesion. The etiology of the intractable plantar keratosis must be looked at in terms of a structural defect or abnormal function causing the lesion to arise. Both abnormal function and structural defect may appear together. Structural defects which cause intractable plantar keratosis are such things as enlarged metatarsal heads, enlarged metatarsal condyles, plantar flexed metatarsals, abnormally long metatarsals, abnormally shaped sesamoids, foreign bodies, and degenerative changes of the metatarsal heads. Some of the biomechanical considerations we will speak about causing intractable plantar keratomas are abnormal pronation, dorsiflexed toes, atrophy of the plantar fat pad and displacement of the plantar fat pad.

The surgical procedures being performed in the United States today for intractable plantar keratosis range from the excision of the lesion to the plantar condylectomies, to metatarsal head resections, to osteotomies performed at every level on the metatarsal shaft; from the head to the neck, to the mid-shaft, to the basal area, to the base itself. It is important before a surgeon undertakes a surgical treatment of intractable plantar keratosis, to understand the function of this specific metatarsal in relationship to the mid-tarsal joint and the mid-tarsal joint's relationship to the sub-talar joint. It is important to take the total relationship of the foot to the leg, the leg to the knee, and the knee to the hip. Many patients present plantar keratosis which readily can be controlled by good orthotic care. In many instances, plantar lesions which had been intractable for years and have had conservative palliation performed, have surgical indications which do not necessitate the usual orthotic control before considering surgery. There are those cases where the etiology is only a structural defect and surgery is the treatment of choice with or without orthotic control. Most plantar lesions are painful, as we will see in this section, due to the shearing force caused by mechanical malalignment which then creates an adventitious bursitis plantar to the metatarsal head. The patients usually present to our offices painful excrescences which are either unsightly and painful, or present burning and frank pain from the surrounding inflammed tissues and underlying bursal sacs. The purpose of this section is not to discuss the total study of biomechanics but rather to narrow the topic to discuss the mechanical changes, commonly causing forefoot intractable lesions. The lesion itself must undergo a good differential diagnosis which should include shearing callus, true plantar lesions such as verruca plantaris, inclusion cysts, foreign body reaction, etc. The surgery is but one means of re-aligning certain structures in the relationship to function, but yet the abnormality which created the lesion to begin with must be controlled by means of an orthotic. Most structural deformities respond well to surgery and/or accommodative orthotics. If the lesions are truly biomechanical in etiology, then functional control with or without surgery usually presents favorable results. An orthotic may be either a functional orthotic as used for a shearing callus, made out of Rohadur, or an accommodative orthotic as used for atrophy of the planter fat pad, made out of a softer accommodative material such as "Molo" and leather. It must be remembered that lesions do present themselves with both an abnormal function and a structural defect portion of the deformity and of course the treatment is then a combination of control and surgery.

Gait Cycle

The gait cycle in its relationship to foot function must be thoroughly understood by the surgeon who is discussing the surgical correction of plantar keratotic lesions. The walking cycle consists of the stance phase of one foot, including the double weight bearing period, and the swing phase of the same leg. The weight bearing period, or stance phase, comprises approximately a 5% variation, 65% of the entire cycle. Much in terms of the mechanics of the patients' presenting complaint, foot function can be determined by asking the patient to walk barefooted and observing the gait pattern. Mann and Inman, in 1964, reported on the phasic activities of muscles during the gait cycle. Wright, in 1964, reported on his studies pertaining to the subtalar and ankle joint complex during the gait cycle. It must be understood that the gait cycle is broken up into three distinct intervals. The first interval being that which extends from heel strike to the foot becoming flat, the second interval occurs at the period that the foot becomes flat and with the body passing over the foot, the third interval extends from the moment the heel rises to toe off. The duration of the second interval is approximately twice as long as the first or third interval. During the course of the gait cycle, the examiner must watch not only the rotational changes of the extremity, but should create a system of examining the subtalar motion during the heel contact and stance phase and then the mid-tarsal joint during stance phase and toe off. The gait cycle should show the heel contact and the examiner should evaluate this as to whether there is a sustained heel contact, no visible early heel off which would indicate an equinus deformity. He must also look to see if the heel stays inverted in relationship to the leg, if it pronates, or if there is excessive pronation noted. We shall discuss the various subtalar deformities later in the chapter.

Common Rearfoot Deformities

The most common deformity noted in the patient with plantar hyperkeratotic lesions is the rearfoot varus deformity. The subtalar joint should be examined to ascertain whether or not the calcaneus is in an inverted position in relationship to the leg. For definition purposes, a rearfoot varus occurs when the sagittal plane of the posterior surface and the plantar surface of the calcaneus are inverted to the weight bearing surface, the subtalar joint is in the neutral position and the body is standing in the angle and base of gait. The rearfoot varus can either be a compensated type or an uncompensated type deformity. The uncompensating rearfootvarus deformity is not as common as the compensated subtalar varus deformity. The rearfoot varus deformity naturally causes the midtarsal joint to remain in a more locked position. Patients presenting this deformity usually have a tendency to sprain their ankle repeatedly or have instability at the ankle and subtalar joint areas. These patients have presenting lesions under the 5th metatarsal head area with large plantar and plantar -lateral lesions with an accompanying Tailor's bunion. A compensated rearfoot varus deformity is usually shown when sufficient subtalar joint pronation is available. A rearfoot varus deformity can be completely compensated by the eversion of the calcaneus until its sagittal plane becomes vertical and the entire plantar surface of the foot comes to rest upon the floor. Such a condition as this is referred to as a totally compensated rearfoot varus. Of course there are variations of this type of compensation. The compensation or the effect of such compensation causes a great amount of shear on the plantar surface of the foot. This of course sets the stage for initiation of plantar intractable lesions.

The Equinus Foot

The term equinus in the literature is usually referred to as a drop foot, but most of our modern biomechanics today refers to a lack of dorsiflexion at the ankle joint as an equinus deformity. Usually the equinus foot is classified according to the etiology which presents itself. The equinus foot is of extreme importance because of its ramification on total foot function. As we said before, in a classic equinus deformity naturally we see an early heel off which loads the forefoot and creates a stress factor because of the force going through the ball of the foot. As we know today, the equinus foot is responsible for the break-down of foot function when it presents itself. The compensations for an equinus foot is usually done with abnormal subtalar joint pronation and possibly midtarsal joint pronation to permit the calcaneus to contact the floor during the early portion of the stance phase of gait. When the foot is totally uncompensated there is really no heel contact and the forefoot bares all the weight during the stance phase. This gait usually is unstable and has small apropulsive steps. In the partially compensated equinus foot, the midtarsal joint generally remains locked and little or no dorsiflexion is achieved by abnormal pronation; this causes subsequent subluxation of the midtarsal joint. Of course in gait, the heel does not evert to the floor. However, shearing calluses beneath the second metatarsal head are usually seen and other lesions along the lesser metatarsal heads can be seen also. The compensated equinus foot is usually seen with abnormal pronation of the subtalar and midtarsal joint to permit the foot to contact the floor and it allows the tibia to angulate 10 degrees to the floor at mid-stance. In other words, the foot compensated by pronating so much at the midtarsal and subtalar joint areas, that the foot is able to dorsiflex sufficiently to compensate for the equinus deformity presenting itself. This foot is extremely flat and the rearfoot is seen to be maximally everted to the floor and to the forefoot. There is severe plantar keratosis formed in this type of foot. The patient also has severe arch pain, leg and back pain. The equinus foot must be recognized prior to treating intractable keratosis so that if indeed the foot is not controllable, with orthotics due to the equinus deformity, the problem of the rearfoot must be tackled to allow proper control of the patient. During the course of the subsequent chapters in this text, we will be able to see why certain procedures can be performed in light of an equinus deformity with rather good success, because the bone is raised high by way of osteoclasis procedures, but yet the complication of allowing the metatarsal to be raised high as we will see in subsequent chapters, is not always worth the surgical exercise, because the patient does develop transfer lesions inspite of the surgery.

Forefoot Varus Deformities

Forefoot varus deformity is a deformity in which the plantar plane of the forefoot is inverted relative to the plantar plane of the rearfoot when the subtalar joint is in its neutral position and the forefoot is pronated to its maximum. The forefoot varus deformity is usually assumed to be an ontogenetic deformity, relating to the lack of valgus rotation of the head and neck of the talus, relative to the body of the talus. It is usually assumed that the lack of valgus rotation at the head and neck of the talus results in the varus positioning of the first ray. The forefoot varus deformity is probably one of the most common midtarsal joint deformities seen, in relationship to intractable plantar keratosis. Again the forefoot varus deformity can either be uncompensated or compensated. In the uncompensated forefoot varus deformity, the subtalar joint motion does not allow the medial aspect of the forefoot to come to the ground. In the compensated forefoot varus deformity, the forefoot varus position causes compensatory subtalar joint pronation. This is because the reactive gravitational force from the floor would predominate against the lateral side of the foot if the subtalar joint tried to supinate back toward its netural position. The midtarsal joint is unlocked, allowing a greater range of motion of the forefoot when the rearfoot joint compensates. The first and fifth rays become subluxed and hypermobile producing a wide variety of forefoot symptoms. The forefoot shows a multitude of plantar lesions usually with the greater degree of hypermobility of the first metatarsal, the sub-second lesion becomes clinically apparent. The inverted forefoot position causes a sub 5th lesion and tailor bunion formation. The condition of forefoot varus must be recognized and controlled postoperatively or the existence of transfer lesions after individual surgical procedures will be imminent. The presence of plantar keratomas in this type of deformity is usually aggrevated by the activity of the patient, the weight of the patient, the circulation of the patient, the skin texture, and the absence of the plantar fat pad. In relationship to plantar keratomas in a patient who has a forefoot varus deformity, he also will usually be seen with a tendency towards a hallux abducto valgus bunion and will also be seen with dislocated digits and midtarsal joint subluxations.

Forefoot Valgus

The forefoot valgus deformity in its relationship to plantar lesions is defined as an ontogenetic deformity where the head and neck of the talus remains everted in relationship to the body of the talus. The plantar aspect of the ball of the foot is seen to be everted relative to the bisection of the calcaneus when the subtalar joint is in its neutral position and the midtarsal joint is maximally pronated. The forefoot must be evaluated to the point where the surgeon must identify whether or not the plantar flexed 1st metatarsal is indeed just a plantarflexed first ray with an accompanying forefoot varus or the presenting deformity is indeed an eversion deformity of the midtarsal joint totally. This type of rigid forefoot valgus deformity or a rigid plantar flexed first ray usually presents a sub first lesion usually under the tibial sesamoid area and this is the type of lesion, surgeons for many years have removed the tibial sesamoid bone for and have found themselves getting into hallux valgus deformities, following the surgical procedure. Again the mechanics of the foot can not be overlooked in the treatment of plantar hyperkeratotic lesions. The patient with this type of deformity with plantar lesions under the tibial sesamoid area, is usually a deeply enucleated lesion with large bursal sacs around the lesion. This deformity can be compensated or uncompensated; the compensation of this deformity is usually seen in the subtalar joint because it becomes inverted so that the foot may become flat against the transverse plane, or that the subtalar joint becomes inverted to compensate for the eversion deformity of the midtarsal joint. One observes a patient with a forefoot valgus in gait, there is a strong tendency to see that it appears to have a normal foot to leg function. Further questioning of this type of patient would reveal that they are unstable at times and have a tendency towards lateral ankle sprains. There is definitely a clinical tendency towards seeing keratomas under the second and third metatarsal heads with eventual Tailors bunion formation and a tendency towards dorsal dislocation of the lesser digits, because of the nature of this foot. Usually the patient with a first ray deformity or a forefoot valgus deformity, shows a tendency towards a very high arched foot with a displacement of the plantar fat pad which usually gives rise to large isolated lesions under the metatarsal head due to the displacement and the fantastic force going through this area of the foot.

Summary

The discussion of mechanics and their relationship to specific intractable plantar keratotic lesions can not be complete unless one becomes a student of biomechanics and understands the total mechanical picture of foot to leg function. In this short chapter as we said in the beginning, it is impossible to do justice to the science of biomechanics, only to shed some light on the possible clinical syndromes, which helped to produce these intractable lesions. The control of the mechanical deformity must be undertaken by the surgeon after the procedure of choice is performed. It is ludicrous to believe that one can do a good piece of surgical carpentry on the operating table and not control the forces which gave rise to the problem in the first place.

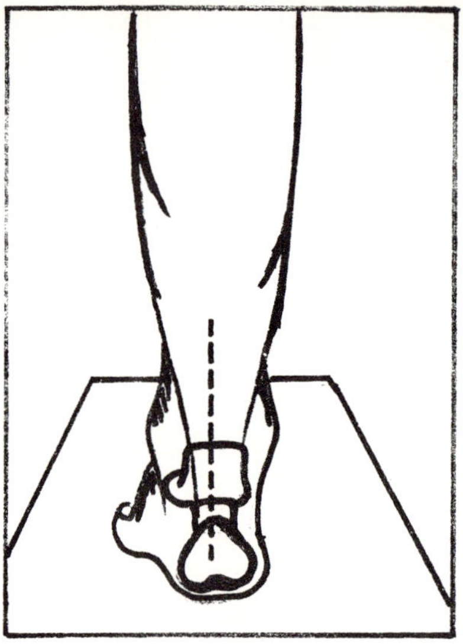

FIGURE 1
NORMAL

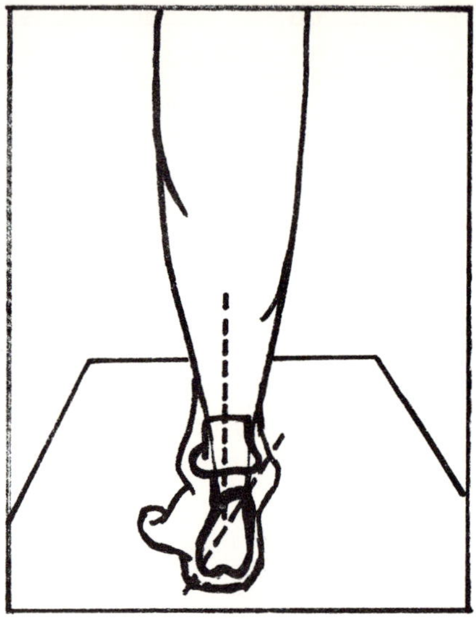

FIGURE 2
UNCOMPENSATED
SUBTALAR VARUS

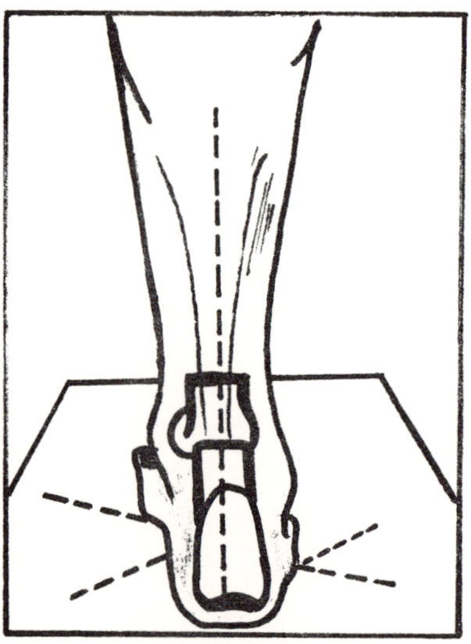

FIGURE 3
UNCOMPENSATED
FOREFOOT VARUS

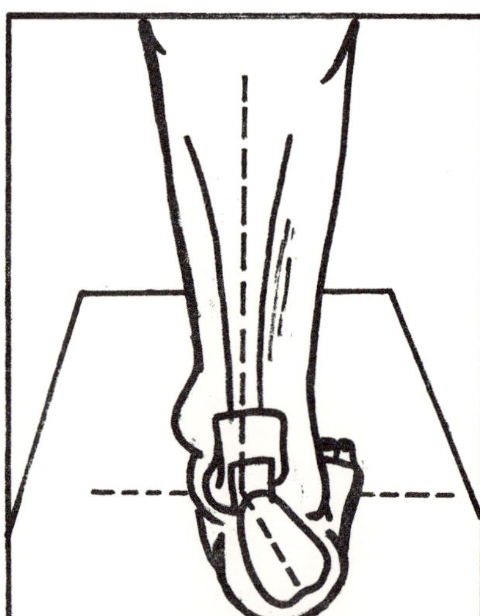

FIGURE 4
COMPENSATED
FOREFOOT VARUS

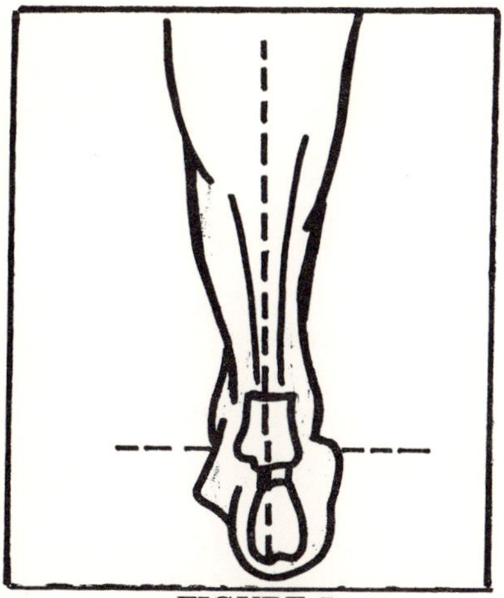

FIGURE 5
UNCOMPENSATED
FOREFOOT VALGUS

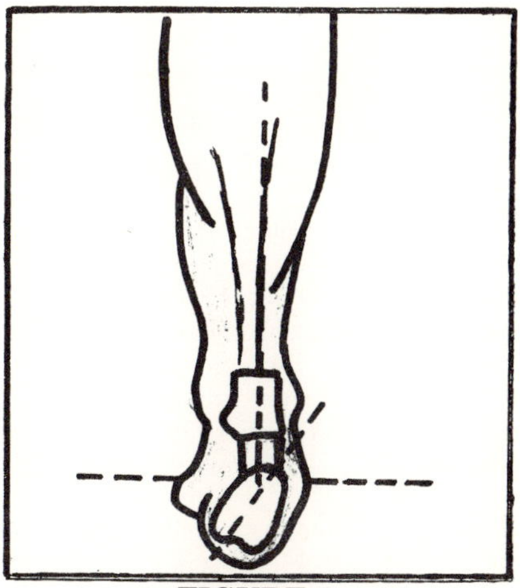

FIGURE 6
COMPENSATED
FOREFOOT VALGUS

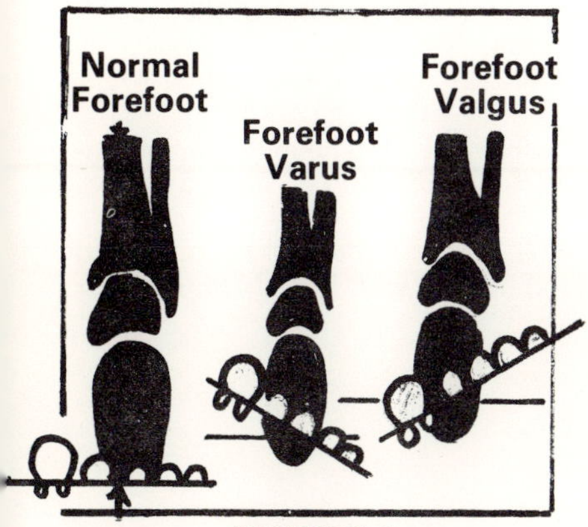

FIGURE 7
SUMMARY OF
MID-TARSAL DEFORMITIES

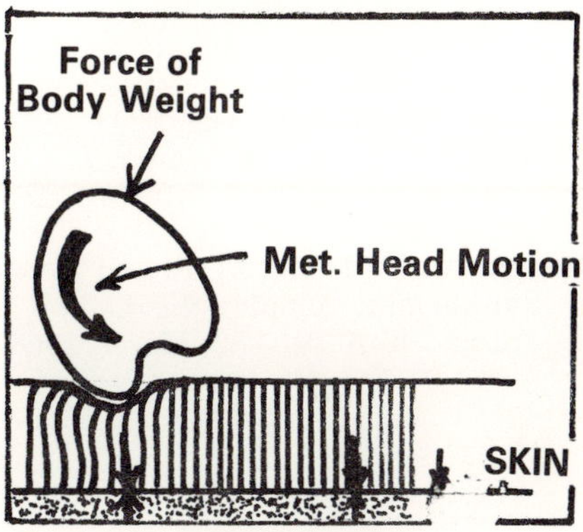

FIGURE 8
METATARSAL SHEARING
AN EXAMPLE OF
CALLOUS FORMATION

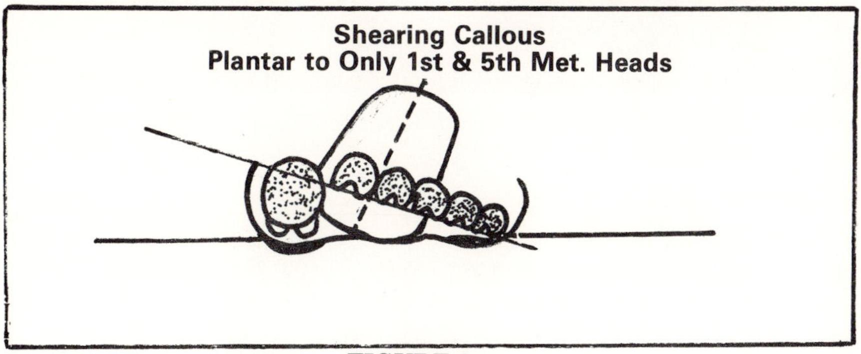

FIGURE 9
Shearing callous plantar to only 1st and 5th metatarsal heads. Seen with supinated subtalar joint due to: Forefoot Valgus; plantarflexed 1st ray; spastic peroneus longus

Bibliography

Close, R. J. and Inman, V. T.: *The Action of the Subtalar Joint,* Prosthetic Devices Research Project, Institute of Engineering Research, University of California, Berkeley, Series II, Issue 24, May 1953.

Close, R. J. and Inman, V. T.: *The Action of the Ankle Joint,* Prosthetic Devices Research Project, Institute of Engineering Research, University of California, Berkeley, Series II, Issue 22, April 1952.

Cunningham, D. M.: *Components of floor reactions during walking.* Prosthetic Devices Research Project, Institute of Engineering Research, University of California, Berkeley, Series II, Issue 14, Berkeley, The Project, Nov. 1950.

Elftman, H.: Forces and Energy Changes in the Leg During Walking, *Am. J. Phys.,* February 1939.

Elftman, H.: Transvere Tarsal Joint and Its Control, *Clinical Orthopedics,* **16**:42.

Hicks, J. H.: Mechanics of the Foot: I. The Joints, *Jr. of Anat.,* **87**:345-357, 1953.

Hicks, J. H.: Mechanics of the Foot - II: The Plantar Aponeurosis and the Arch, *Jr. of Anat.,* **88**:25-31, 1954.

Hicks, J. H.: Mechanics of the Foot: IV: Action of Muscles on the Foot in Standing, *Acta Anat.,* **27**:180-192.

Mann, R. and Inman, V. T.: Phasic activity of intrinsic muscles of the foot, *J. Bone Joint Surg.,* **46-A**:469-481, April 1964.

Manter, J. T.: Movements of the subtalar and transverse tarsal joints, *Anat. Rec.,* **80**:397-410, Aug. 1941.

Saunders, J. B. deC. M., Inman, V. T. and Eberhart, H. D.: The major determinants in normal and pathological gait, *J. Bone Joint Surg.,* **35-A**:543-558, July 1953.

Wright, D. G., Desai, M. E. and Henderson, B. S.: Action of the subtalar and ankle-joint complex during the stance phase of walking, *J. Bone Joint Surg.,* **46-A**:361-382, March 1964.

B. Radiographic Examination and Evaluation

The radiological evaluation of the foot that has an intractable plantar keratoma is extremely important in that it affords the physician the necessary facts to confirm his clinical impressions and, in many instances, to understand the etiology for the particular lesion. One must realize that the X-ray is only a specialized test and can not be utilized by itself in making the diagnosis and determining the treatment to be rendered. The clinical examination of the lesion, the foot, the extremity, and the patient, is the most important aspect in making the diagnosis and formulating a treatment plan.

There are numerous radiographic views which can be taken in order to evaluate this condition; however the following views are generally sufficient — I. the anterior-posterior view of the foot; II. the lateral view of the foot; and III. the axial view of the foot. Before discussing the particular views there are several general factors which should be mentioned. First of all, the X-rays must be taken in the patient's angle and base of gait in order to assure more reliable information and in order to be able to reproduce the approximate position of the foot in subsequent X-rays at a later date for comparison. Second, by labeling the lesion with a lead marker prior to taking the X-ray views, one can more accurately determine the location of the lesion in relationship to the osseous structures. This is not to say that in all instances can one find a cause-effect relationship.

I. Anterior-Posterior (A.P.) View:

This view will give the physician perhaps the most information in evaluating the intractable plantar keratoma. The following is a list of those facts which can be ascertained by examining this X-ray view:

1. The relationship of the lesion that was labeled with a lead marker to the metatarsal heads.
2. The degenerative changes which may have occurred at the level of the metatarsal-phalangeal joint area.
3. The presence or absence of a foreign body in this area.
4. The parabola of the metatarsals. Many times an abnor-

mally long metatarsal or abnormally short metatarsals may be the etiology of the intractable plantar keratoma.

5. The size of the metatarsal heads. Congenitally or following trauma a metatarsal head may be abnormally large or malformed which could be the etiology of the plantar lesion.
6. The position of the toes in relationship to the metatarsal-phalangeal joints. Dorsiflexed toes force the metatarsals plantar thereby possibly producing the plantar lesion.
7. The position and shape of the hallucal sesamoids.
8. The presence or absence of accessory sesamoid bones plantar to the metatarsal heads.
9. The presence or absence of abnormal pronatory changes and osseous adaptive changes.

II. Lateral View:

The following is a list of those facts which can be ascertained by examining this X-ray view:

1. The sagittal position of the first metatarsal (dorsiflexed, plantarflexed).
2. The position and shape of the tibial sesamoid bone of the hallux.
3. The relationship of the toes to the metatarsals. As mentioned previously, dorsiflexion of the toes plantarflexes the metatarsals and could be the etiology of the intractable plantar keratoma.
4. The amount of soft tissue density beneath the metatarsal heads. In the older patient and/or when the toes are dorsally contracted, the plantar fat pad becomes atrophied and/or displaced anteriorly.
5. The presence or absence of abnormal pronatory changes and adaptive osseous changes.

III. Axial View:

Over the past several years the axial view of the foot which is a plantar view of the metatarsal heads has become quite popular. More importantly, since the advent of the axial view positioning device, this view has become more helpful in evaluating the intractable plantar keratoma. However, in examining this view one must understand the apparent normal relationship of one metatarsal to another that this positioning device creates. Since the first and fifth metatarsals are the most mobile, the device causes them to be the most plantarflexed of all metatarsals. The fourth is next, followed by the third metatarsal then the second metatarsal. Therefore in the so-called normal foot on the positioning device the second metatarsal head would appear to be the most dorsal and the first and fifth the most plantar. Consequently if one should view the second metatarsal head on the same plane as the first metatarsal head it would be considered plantarflexed even though it was not below the plane of all metatarsal heads. Remember, one must evaluate the metatarsal heads in their relative position to one another when the foot is placed on the axial view positioning device. Without the device one can not really determine whether one metatarsal is truly plantarflexed in relationship to another because of the many variables which are encountered in positioning the foot for this view without the device. The following is a list of those facts which can be ascertained by examining this special view taken on the positioning device:

1. The shape and position of the hallucal sesamoids.
2. The presence or absence of accessory sesamoid bones plantar to the metatarsal heads.
3. The shape of the plantar condyles of the metatarsals.
4. The size of the metatarsal heads and their condition.
5. The relative position of the metatarsal heads to one another. A plantarflexed metatarsal is a common etiological factor producing the plantar lesion.
6. The amount of soft tissue density beneath the metatarsal heads.

In conclusion one must remember that the X-ray is only an adjunct to the clinical examination. In no way should it be utilized by itself to make the diagnosis and to determine the treatment plan. As physicians we treat patients, not X-rays.

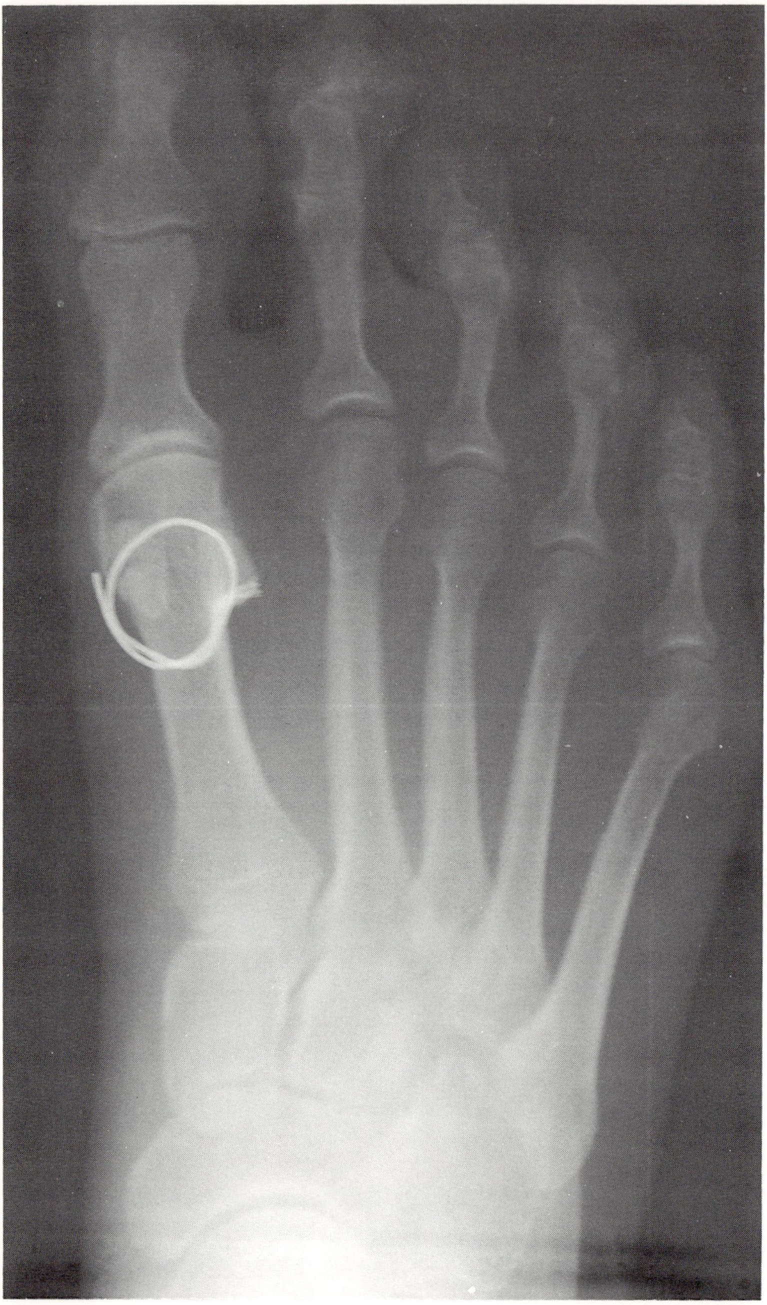

FIGURE 1

An example of an Intractable Plantar Keratoma under the tibial sesamoid, with marker.

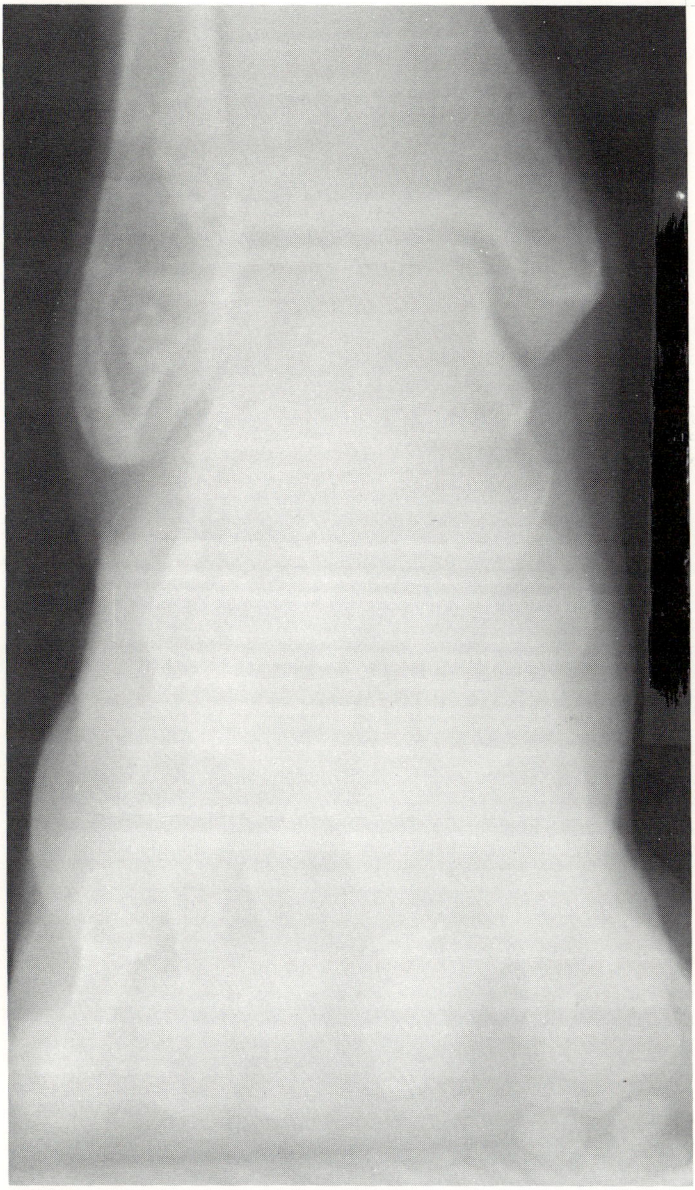

FIGURE 2

An example of an axial X-ray, with marker.

Bibliography

Downey, Margaret A. and Dorothy, Wayne, L.: A radiographic technique to demonstrate the plantar aspect of the forefoot in stance. *J.A.P.A.*, **59**(4), 1969.

Sgarlato, T. E.: *Compendium of Podiatric Biomechanics.* California College of Podiatric Medicine. San Francisco, 1971.

SECTION III

SURGICAL PROCEDURES

A. First Metatarsal IPK

The intractable plantar keratoma located beneath the first metatarsal head must be carefully evaluated clinically and radiographically to determine the exact etiology. This section will deal with the various surgical procedures which can be employed depending upon the etiology of the lesion.

1. Tibial Sesamoidectomy

This procedure is the excision of the tibial sesamoid bone which is located beneath the first metatarsal head. In performing it one should take certain precautionary measures in order to prevent the occurence of hallux deformity postoperatively due to the imbalance created at the first metatarsal-phalangeal joint.

Preoperative Signs

1. A well delineated intractable plantar keratoma plantar to the tibial sesamoid.
2. Atrophy of the plantar fat pad may be present.
3. Prominent tibial sesamoid bone upon direct palpation is usually present.
4. Hallux deformity may be present.
5. Hallux limitus or hallux rigidus may be present.
6. Hallux extensus may be present.

Preoperative Symptoms

1. Pain in and around the first metatarsal-phalangeal joint during ambulation with or without foot gear.
2. Pain with direct pressure to the plantar lesion.
3. Inability to move the hallux adequately may be a complaint.
4. History of trauma to the area of the first metatarsal head may be obtained.
5. History of arthritis may be obtained.
6. Inability to wear certain types of shoes may be a complaint.

Biomechanical Evaluation

1. A forefoot valgus deformity has proven to be detrimental to the long term prognosis.
2. This procedure can be performed in the presence of uncontrollable pronatory forces.
3. A plantarflexed first ray has proven to be detrimental to the long term prognosis.
4. Some form of an orthotic, either functional or accomodative, is needed postoperatively.

Preoperative X-ray Evaluation

1. Irregularity of the tibial sesamoid is usually seen.
2. Enlargement of the tibial sesamoid may be present on an axial view of the foot.
3. A bi-partite sesamoid may be present.
4. An abnormal position of the tibial sesamoid may be present.
5. A fractured tibial sesamoid may be present.
6. A fused tibial sesamoid to the metatarsal head may be present.
7. Arthritis of the first metatarsal-phalangeal joint may be present.

Surgical Procedure

The avoidance of some of the complications which relate to sesamoid surgery requires much surgical care and detailed considerations of the anatomy of the entire first metatarsal-phalangeal joint and its periarticular structures. The following are various surgical complications and methods presented by E.D. McGlamry to avoid them. It must be remembered that a tibial sesamoidectomy weakens the flexor hallucis brevis muscle by removing a fulcrum for the tendon. It also leaves a somewhat loose tendon when the mass of the sesamoid has been removed. In essence, one has lengthened the tibial tendon slip of the flexor hallucis brevis. With these considerations in mind some provisions must be made to prevent the dorsal structures from overwhelming the plantar tendons and capsule resulting in a cock-up hallux or a hallux abductus, especially in a foot which already has a certain degree of instability. The following ways to prevent complications need not always be taken. Careful evaluation of the foot and the stability of the first metatarsal-phalangeal joint will dictate the amount of prevention one must undertake.

In the case of a tibial sesamoidectomy for an intractable plantar keratoma in an unstable foot due to pronatory forces and a deviated first metatarsal-phalangeal joint the following should be performed to prevent a hallux deformity. A dorsal linear skin incision is made just medial to the extensor hallucis longus tendon and parallel to it over the first metatarsal-phalangeal joint. By sharp and blunt dissection the extensor longus is isolated and lengthened depending upon the deformity of the hallux. Care should be taken to lengthen it only the amount that is required. A tenotomy of the extensor hallucis brevis tendon should then be performed. This is important since it is inserted almost directly opposite to the insertion of the flexor hallucis brevis tendon from which the tibial sesamoid is to be removed. If there is a moderate to severe dorsal contracture it is wise to perform a dorsal capsulotomy of the metatarsal-phalangeal joint. Then, by careful blunt and sharp dissection, the medial aspect of the joint is freed of all subcutaneous tissue down to the plantar aspect of the capsule. By having an assistant apply pressure on the plantar aspect of metatarsal head in a dorsal direction one can free this subcutaneous tissue from the medial aspect of the joint more easily, especially the plantar aspect. A longitudinal incision is made along the plantar aspect of the joint medially (Fig. 1). Also from the medial side of the joint capsule an inverted "V" portion of the capsule is removed. The base of the "V" lies continuous with the longitudinal incision in the joint. The apex of the "V" points dorsally and ends about the dorsal-medial margin on the side of the first metatarsal head. Reflecting the capsule which has been incised makes it quite easy to remove the tibial sesamoid. It should be shelled from the dorsal aspect of the medial tendon slip in which it is invested being careful not to severe the long flexor tendon. One must incise the tibial sesamoid ligament, the plantar tibial sesamoid ligament, and the intersesamoid ligament in order to totally remove the tibial sesamoid bone. The area should be flushed well and inspected to make sure the long flexor was not severed and that there were no fragments of bone left in the area. The wedge shaped incision and the longitudinal incision in the joint capsule are then closed with absorbable sutures. Removal of the wedge of capsule does much to minimize the tendency toward developing hallux abductus. It also strengthens the tibial side of the joint and prevents abnormal extension of the proximal phalanx. The subcutaneous tissue and skin are closed in the usual manner. If you do not feel that the extensor tendon has to be corrected then you could use a curved medial skin incision over the first metatarsal-phalangeal joint. The area is dressed in the usual sterile manner with the hallux being splinted if possible in its normal position.

If the plantar lesion was extremely fibrotic and not too large then it should probably be excised. It has been our experience that even after removing the offending piece of bone the lesion remains if it was originally fibrotic and deep. With time it may disappear; however the patient is usually quite disturbed to find the lesion still present many months following surgery. The lesion can be ellipsed and the tissues approximated using a non-absorbable suture. Silk seems to work quite well and is tolerated by the patient during ambulation better than nylon or steel. Several drops of a non-repository steroid such as dexamethasone are placed in the site of the tibial sesamoid excision. This has been found to reduce the postoperative inflammatory phase and reduces the patients discomfort.

Postoperative Management

The hallux is splinted for 3 to 4 weeks and the patient is encouraged to begin ambulating 24 hours postoperatively. If the plantar lesion was ellipsed the patient is kept non-weight bearing for 2 weeks or accomodative padding is constructed in the post-operative shoe to eliminate pressure from the plantar surgical site. The dressings are changed at weekly intervals and the sutures are removed approximately 14 days postoperatively. The plantar sutures, if any were used, are usually not removed until 21 days postoperatively. The patient can usually return to normal foot gear in 4 to 6 weeks. An orthotic of some type is constructed for the patient when he can utilize normal foot gear.

Advantages

1. It eliminates the internal etiological factor.
2. It is not a technically difficult surgical procedure.
3. The postoperative disability for the patient is minimal.
4. It may increase the range of motion of the first metatarsal-phalangeal joint postoperatively.

5. It preserves the stability of the first metatarsal-phalangeal joint if performed properly.

Disadvantages

1. It may increase a hallux abductus deformity if precautionary measures are not employed.
2. The range of motion of the first metatarsal-phalangeal joint may be decreased.
3. If the flexor hallucis longus tendon is severed and not repaired a hallux extensus and/or a cock-up hallux will occur.
4. This procedure will not eliminate the plantar lesion or symptoms if the sesamoid was not the etiological factor.

A. This is a medial view of the first metatarso-phalangeal joint showing the investment of the sesamoid in the tendon of the flexor hallucis brevis and the type of capsulotomy employed to remove the sesamoid. Note how the entire sesamoid bone is invested in tendon and/or capsule except for the dorsal surface which articulates with the plantar aspect of the first metatarsal head. The "V" shaped piece of capsule which is excised is to help prevent a postoperative hallux abducto-valgus.

B. This is a medial view of the first metatarso-phalangeal joint showing the capsule reflected to expose two deep ligaments; the proximal one must be severed to remove the sesamoid.

C. This is a medial view showing the ligaments and tendon that are deep to the capsule. The capsule is not shown in this drawing. (1) the medial collateral ligament (2) the plantar tibial sesamoid ligament (3) the tendon of the flexor hallucis brevis muscle and (4) the tibial sesamoid ligament. In order to remove the tibial sesamoid bone one must sever the tibial sesamoid ligament, the plantar tibial sesamoid ligament, the medial tendon of the flexor hallucis brevis muscle, and the intersesamoid ligament which is not shown on these drawings.

D. This is the medial view of the first metatarso-phalangeal joint capsule after removal of the sesamoid and closure of the capsulotomy.

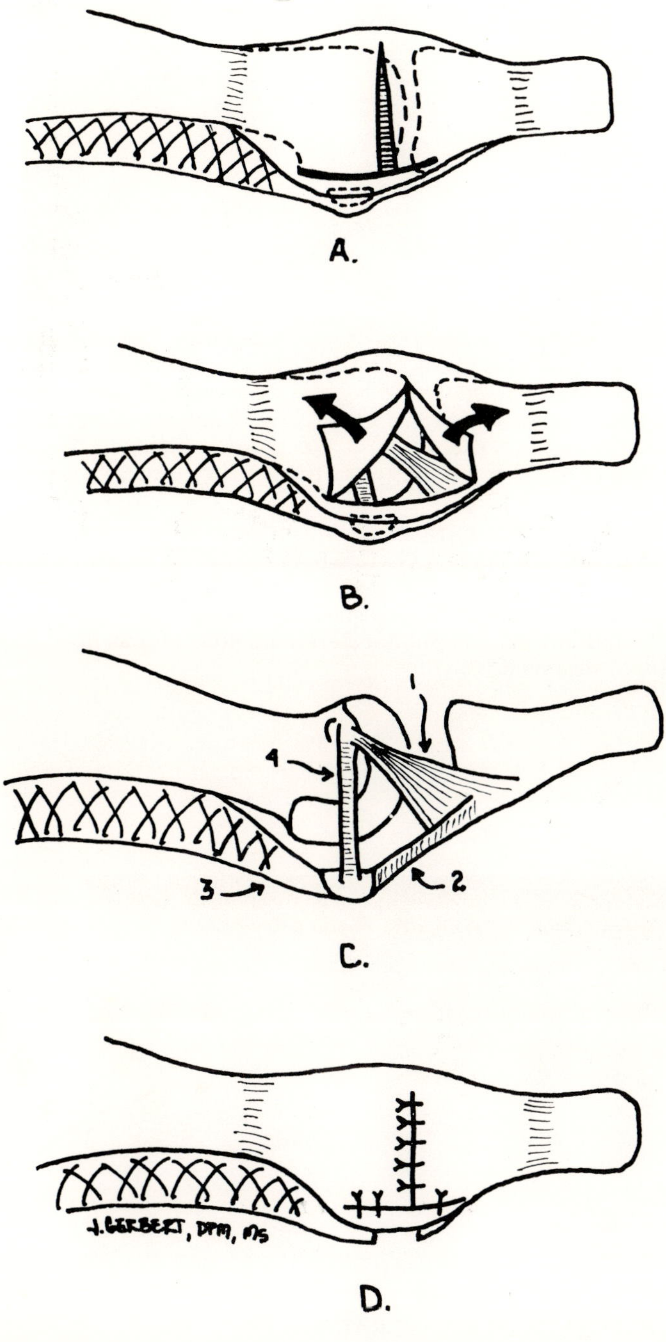

FIGURE 1
TIBIAL SESAMOIDECTOMY

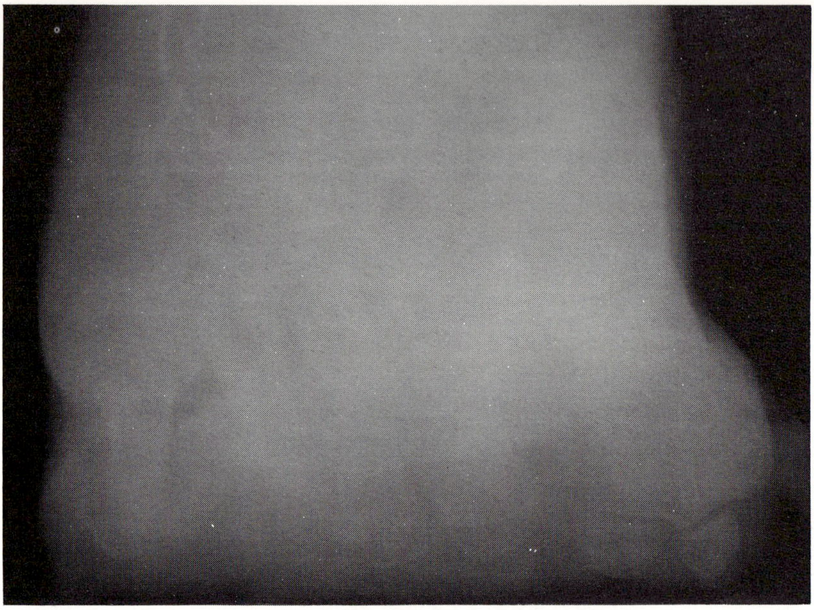

FIGURE 2
PREOPERATIVE AXIAL X-RAY

This is an axial view demonstrating the deformed tibial sesamoid. Clinically, the patient had an intractable plantar keratoma plus a bursa directly under the tibial sesamoid.

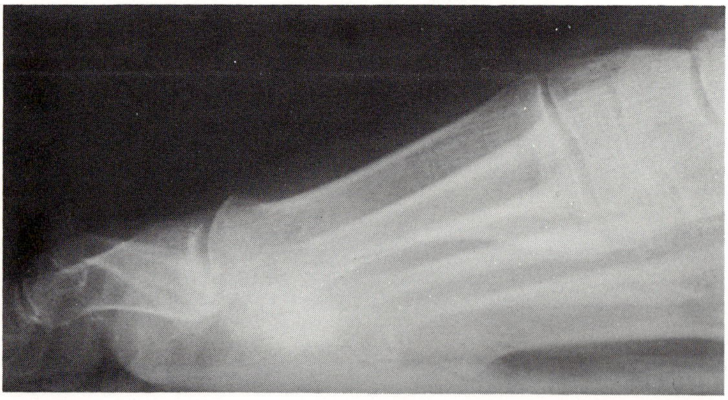

FIGURE 3
PREOPERATIVE LATERAL X-RAY

This is a lateral view showing that the first metatarsal is not plantarflexed, which must be considered before deciding to remove the sesamoid as the causative factor.

2. Fibular Sesamoidectomy

This procedure is the excision of the fibular sesamoid bone and is usually performed in conjunction with a bunionectomy procedure. On rare occasions however one finds it necessary to excise it as a solitary procedure in order to eliminate an intractable plantar keratoma. It is usually the result of trauma to the sesamoid bone or severe degenerative arthritis of the bone.

Preoperative Signs

1. A well delineated intractable plantar keratoma to the fibular sesamoid.
2. Atrophy of the plantar fat pad may be present.
3. Prominent fibular sesamoid upon direct palpation is usually present.
4. The hallux is usually in normal alignment.
5. A hallux extensus may be present.
6. A decreased range of motion of the first metatarsal-phalangeal joint may be present.

Preoperative Symptoms

1. Pain in and around the first metatarsal-phalangeal joint during ambulation with and without foot gear.
2. Pain with direct pressure to the plantar lesion.
3. Inability to move the hallux adequately may be a complaint.
4. History of trauma to the involved area is usually present.
5. History of arthritis may be obtained in some patients.
6. Inability to wear certain types of shoes may be a complaint.

Biomechanical Evaluation

1. This procedure can be performed in the presence of uncontrollable pronatory forces.
2. Some form of an orthotic either functional or accomodative is needed postoperatively.

Preoperative X-ray Evaluation

1. Irregularity of the fibular sesamoid bone is usually seen.
2. Enlargement of the fibular sesamoid may be present on an axial view of the foot.
3. A bi-partite sesamoid may be present.
4. A fractured fibular sesamoid may be present.
5. The fibular sesamoid bone may be fused to the first metatarsal head.
6. Arthritis of the first metatarsal-phalangeal joint with bony proliferation of the fibular sesamoid may be present.

Surgical Procedure

Keep in mind that the removal of the fibular sesamoid can set up an imbalance of the intrinsic muscles which will affect the first metatarsal-phalangeal joint. However, this usually occurs only when this procedure is performed in conjunction with a bunionectomy. It is in this situation where, after performing a medial capsulotomy and realignment of the tibial sesamoid, one may create a hallux varus, a hallux adductus and/or a cocked-up hallux. In this discussion only the excision of the fibular sesamoid bone as a solitary procedure will be described.

A dorsal linear skin incision is made just lateral to the extensor hallucis longus tendon at the level of the first metatarsal-phalangeal joint. Using sharp and blunt dissection the subcutaneous tissue is freed from the dorsal-lateral aspect of the joint capsule. This dissection is carried down to the floor of the first interspace. Care should be taken to preserve the neurovascular anatomy in this area. Furthermore this dissection should be performed using almost the entire length of the skin incision in order to avoid working through a peep-hole. Using a blunt instrument the fibular sesamoid is palpated. An incision is made parallel and just dorsal to the sesamoid. This incision in the capsule is approximately parallel to the long axis of the first metatarsal. In extends distally to a point just dorsal to the insertion of the adductor hallucis tendon. The scalpel is re-introduced in the same incision and is backed up in the incision until the cutting edge of the blade is just proximal to the sesamoid. The flat edge of the blade is pressed plantarly against the tendon while a short sawing stroke action is begun distally with the instrument. The edge of the sesamoid is encountered as the blade begins to cut between the sesamoid and the tendon fibers. As cutting progresses distally, the blunt edge of the blade is gradually raised so that the cutting edge of the instrument contacts the sesamoid at approximately a 35 to 45 degree angle. In this way the flat edge of the blade retracts the tendon while the cutting edge separates the tendon from the sesamoid. This permits freeing of all the sesamoid attachments with the exception of the intersesamoid ligament. With the hallux flexed and the metatarsal head elevated, the blade can be placed plantar and parallel to the sesamoid bone. The cutting edge of the blade can then be directed against the ligament from underneath. By freeing the proximal aspect of the sesamoid first you can prevent a complication of the sesamoid retracting proximal under the metatarsal after the distal aspect is severed.

You should then inspect the area where the sesamoid was excised to make sure that the long flexor tendon was not severed.

The area should be flushed and the subcutaneous tissues closed in such a manner as to obliterate all dead space. The capsule incision is not closed. The skin is approximated using a nonabsorbable suture material. Several drops of dexamethasone are placed in the site of the fibular excision which helps reduce the postoperative inflammatory reaction and the patients discomfort. If the plantar lesion is well demarcated and quite fibrotic it should be ellipsed in order to give the patient a better postoperative result.

Postoperative Management

The surgical site is dressed in the usual manner for approximately two weeks. The patient is encouraged to begin ambulating 24 hours postoperatively. If the plantar lesion was ellipsed the patient is kept non-weight bearing for 2 weeks or an accomodative pad is constructed in the postoperative shoe to eliminate pressure from the plantar surgical site. The dressings are changed at weekly intervals and the sutures are removed approximately 14 days following surgery. The plantar sutures, if any were used, are usually not removed until 21 days postoperatively. The patient can return to normal foot gear in 3 to 4 weeks. An orthotic of some type is constructed for the patient when he returns to normal foot gear. If the plantar lesion was not ellipsed then the patient should be told that it will take a period of time before the lesion begins resolving. The doctor should definitely keep the lesion reduced during the postoperative recovery phase.

Advantages

1. It eliminates the internal etiological factor.
2. It is not a technically difficult surgical procedure.
3. The postoperative disability for the patient is minimal.
4. It may increase the range of motion of the first metatarsal-phalangeal joint.
5. It may help eliminate a deforming force on the hallux in an unstable foot due to pronatory forces.

Disadvantages

1. This procedure will not eliminate the plantar lesion or symtoms if the fibular sesamoid was not the etiological factor.
2. If the flexor tendon of the hallucis longus was severed and not repaired a hallux extensus or a cocked-up hallux will occur.
3. A hematoma may develop in the first interspace if care is not taken to ligate all bleeders and obliterate all dead space.
4. The range of motion of the first metatarsal-phalangeal joint may be decreased postoperatively.

A. Dorsal view demonstrating the dorsal linear skin incision lateral to the extensor hallucis longus tendon. Only a small portion of the fibular sesamoid is protruding from under the metatarsal head. The first incision in excising the sesamoid is a dorsal linear one just superior to the adductor tendon.

B. This is a medial view showing the hallux plantarflexed and the metatarsal dorsiflexed. This is a useful maneuver in relaxing the flexor hallucis longus tendon in order to prevent severing it and to make it easier to dissect around the sesamoid.

C. This dorsal view shows how retractors can be used to help visualize more of the sesamoid. The medial retractor pulls the metatarsal head medially thereby exposing more of the fibular sesamoid. The sesamoid is freed of its attachments and removed distally.

D. This is a diagram representing the various attachments to the sesamoid and the order in which they should be severed.
   1. Lateral slip of the flexor hallucis brevis
   2. The lateral aspect of the capsule and tendon investment
   3. The plantar fibular sesamoid ligament and tendon of the flexor hallucis brevis
   4. The intersesamoid ligament

   One should leave some tissue at the distal-lateral aspect of the sesamoid bone as shown at the base of the arrow in order for the surgeon to stabilize the sesamoid while dissecting it free without actually clamping onto the bone.

E. This is a frontal plane view of the first metatarsal head showing the following:
   1. Lateral collateral ligament
   2. Fibular sesamoid ligament
   3. Capsule
   4. Adductor tendon dorsal to the transverse metatarsal ligament—the line above this structure represents the initial incision which is shown in A
   5. Plantar fibular sesamoid ligament; and
   6. Flexor hallucis longus tendon

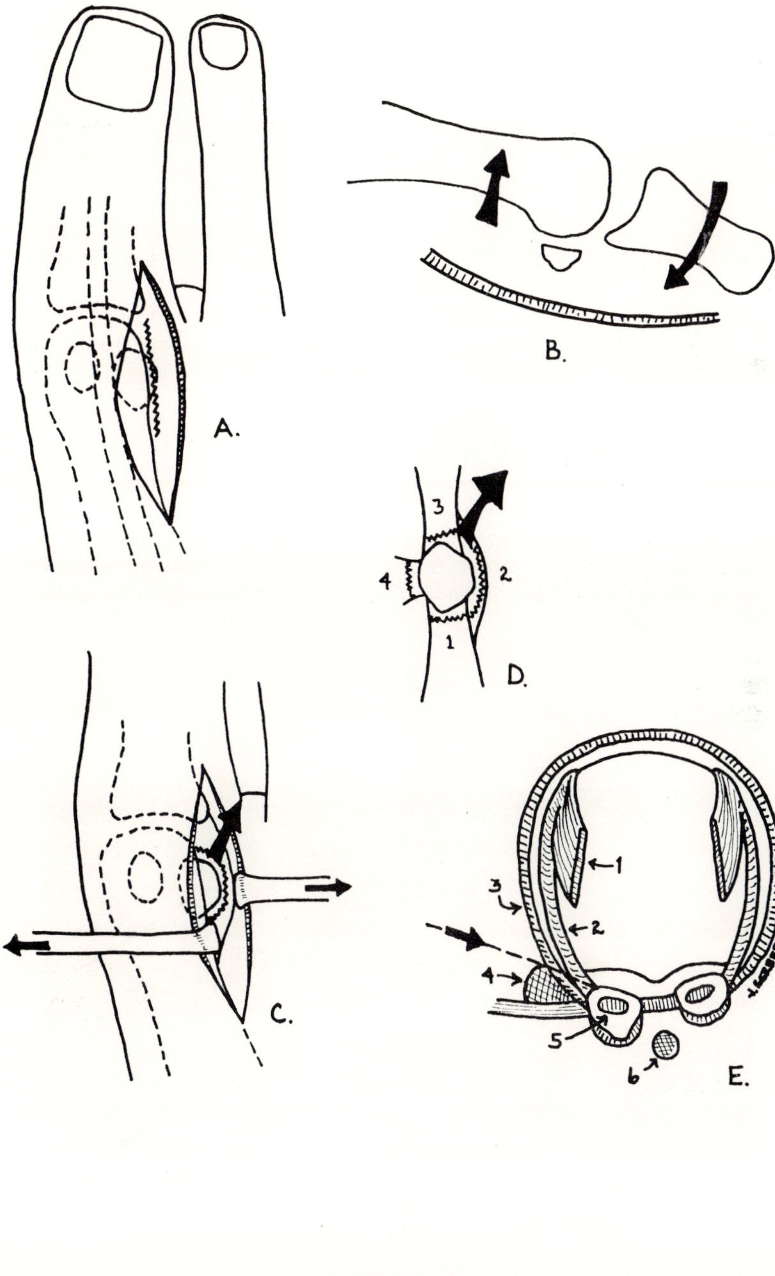

FIGURE 1
FIBULAR SESAMOIDECTOMY

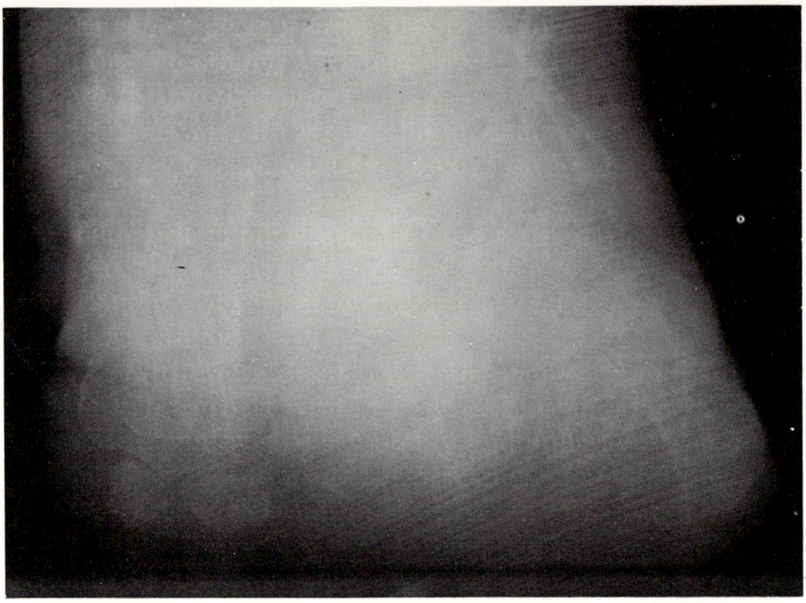

FIGURE 2
PREOPERATIVE AXIAL X-RAY

This is an axial view demonstrating a hypertrophied deformed fibular sesamoid. Note that it is under the metatarsal head bearing weight. Clinically, the patient had an intractable plantar keratoma directly under the fibular sesamoid.

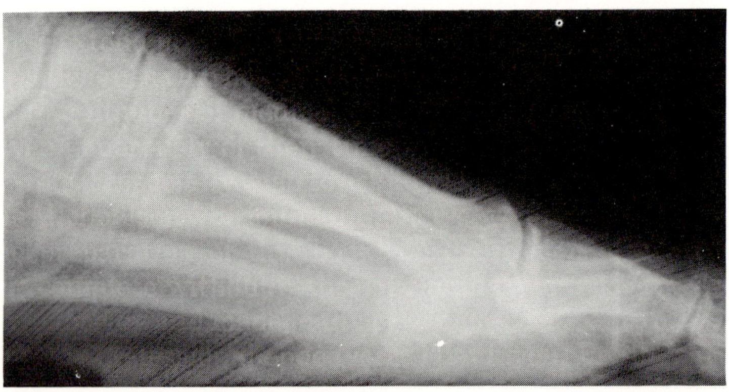

FIGURE 3
PREOPERATIVE LATERAL X-RAY

This is a lateral view showing that the first metatarsal is not plantarflexed. This must be considered before one decides to remove the sesamoid as the causative factor.

3. Dorsal Wedge Osteotomy

This is an osteotomy performed at the proximal portion of the first metatarsal with the base of the wedge dorsal and the apex plantar. By closing this wedge the distal portion of the metatarsal is moved to a more dorsal position. One must be careful not to elevate the metatarsal too high as the motion at the metatarsal-phalangeal joint is decreased as the metatarsal is dorsiflexed. The procedure is utilized for nucleated lesions under the head of the first metatarsal. The sesamoid bones are shown to be normal on the axial view X-ray.

Preoperative Signs

1. An intractable plantar keratoma under the first metatarsal head is present.
2. Atrophy of the plantar fat pad may be present.
3. The tibial sesamoid is not prominent upon direct palpation.
4. An adequate range of motion at the first metatarsal-phalangeal joint must be present.
5. A hallux abducto valgus may be present.
6. A hallux hammertoe may be present.
7. The first metatarsal, when palpated with the foot loaded, is lower than the second metatarsal.
8. A rigid first ray is present.

Preoperative Symptoms

1. Pain plantar to the first metatarsal during ambulation with or without foot gear.
2. Pain exaggerated when wearing high-heeled shoes.
3. Pain exaggerated when walking without shoes on a hard surface.
4. Pain with direct pressure to the keratoma.
5. Inability to wear certain types of foot gear.
6. Medial arch pain or fatigue may be present.

Biomechanical Evaluation

1. A plantar flexed first ray may be present.
2. A total forefoot valgus may be present.
3. The procedure may be performed in the presence of uncontrollable pronatory forces.
4. Postoperative orthotic control should be utilized.

Preoperative X-ray Evaluation

1. A normal tibial sesamoid is present.
2. The first metatarsal appears depressed in relation to the second metatarsal.

3. The first metatarsal may be longer than the second.
4. The epiphysis of the first metatarsal should be closed.
5. The first metatarsal should be of normal bone density.
6. A normal metatarsus primus adductus angle should be present.
7. A hallux abducto-valgus may be present.

Surgical Procedure

The amount of wedge that is necessary to be removed to reduce the deformity should be calculated preoperatively. One may refer to Fig. 1 to determine this calculation.

A four centimeter dorsal linear incision is made over the dorsum of the bone from the metatarsal-cuneiform articulation to the distal one third of the shaft of the metatarsal. By sharp dissection the subcutaneous tissue and deep fascia is incised. The extensor hallucis longus tendon is visualized, freed, and reflected laterally. An incision is made through the periosteum of the metatarsal. A sharp periosteal elevator is used to strip the periosteum from the proximal portion of the metatarsal shaft. Care must be used so that the periosteum is left intact. The metatarsal-cuneiform articulation may now be located so that the site at which the osteotomy will be performed may be determined. Once the osteotomy site is located one is able to plot out the width of the osteotomy. Using a small oscillating blade with power equipment a perpendicular cut is made through the shaft of the metatarsal leaving the plantar cortex in tact. The remainder of the wedge to be removed is then taken from the proximal portion of the bone. Generally the size of this wedge is between three and six millimeters of bone. While stabilizing the proximal segment, the distal portion is dorsiflexed to close the osteotomy. When the site is closed with undue tension, fixation may be obtained. Drill holes are placed proximally and distally to the osteotomy site; two are on the medial aspect of the metatarsal shaft and two on the lateral aspect. A wire loop is constructed and placed in the osteotomy site. A double strand of 28 gauge (2-0) monofilament stainless steel is passed through each hole into the center of the osteotomy site. By pulling the wire loop through the center of the osteotomy site the four wires should be brought dorsally through the osteotomy site. The wires are identified and separated. A hemostat is placed through the proximal wire to grasp the distal wire. The latter wire is brought through the proximal wire and they are twisted to form a union. The proximal wire is then pulled through the holes bringing the distal wire with it. The wires are disengaged so that only a double strand of wire crosses the osteotomy. This is performed on the medial and lateral set of holes. The osteotomy is closed and held in place while the wires are twisted to secure the fixation. See Fig. 2. The periosteum is closed to cover the wire sutures with 3-0 absorbable suture and the subcutaneous tissue is closed with 4-0 absorbable suture. The skin is approximated with 5-0 simple interupted suture or subcuticular suture. The plantar lesion may be excised if it is well demarcated and fibrotic.

Postoperative Management

The patient is placed in a below knee walking cast. Ambulation is allowed 24 to 36 hours following surgery when the cast is dry. The patient is seen at weekly intervals to check the cast. In approximately three weeks the cast may be changed and sutures removed. X-rays should be taken at this time which may reveal early callus formation. It should be noted that if the patient had bilateral procedures, the cast should be changed on separate occasions 48 to 72 hours apart. The cast is reapplied for another 3 weeks. At the end of this time it is removed and the usual physical therapy is begun. An ace bandage and Bevin shoe should be worn for one week to prevent postcast edema. Impressions are taken for the purpose of constructing orthotics for functional control.

Advantages

1. It reduces the primary osseous deformity.
2. The relationship of the first metatarsal to the second metatarsal may be determined during surgery.
3. The height that the first metatarsal may be moved may be controlled.
4. The intrinsic stability of the first metatarsal-phalangeal joint is not disturbed.
5. It may shorten the first metatarsal slightly.
6. The ability to calculate preoperatively the amount of bone needed to be excised to achieve desired correction.

Disadvantages

1. Internal fixation is necessary.
2. Plaster immobilization is required.
3. Prolonged disability and inconvenience for the patient is required.
4. A decrease in motion at the metatarsal-phalangeal joint is possible.
5. Distraction of the ostectomy site is possible, which could result in poor alignment of the metatarsal, creating new symptomatology.
6. Osteoporosis may ensue.
7. Care must be taken to properly use the power equipment to avoid its complications.

These three drawings demonstrate the method for calculating the amount of bone to be removed to reduce the deformity.

A. The first calculation necessary is determining the distance that the metatarsal needs to be raised. One draws a line connecting the plantar aspect of the fifth metatarsal with the sesamoid bones. The new level of the first metatarsal is then estimated and a line is drawn across the ball of the foot. Notice that all metatarsals are not on this line. The third side of the triangle (black arrow) is the distance the first metatarsal is to be raised.

B. The second step is to determine the site of the osteotomy. This is usually 1 cm to 1.5 cm distal to the metatarsal cuneiform articulation. It should be distal to the flair of the metatarsal base. It is now necessary to construct another triangle. One side is the height that the metatarsal will be moved. The other two sides are lines from the osteotomy site to the sesamoid bones in its present position and anticipated position. One can then measure angle Y.

C. Angle Y is then measured on the first metatarsal at the osteotomy site. As the two lines forming this angle transect the superior aspect of the first metatarsal, the width of wedge necessary to move the metatarsal dorsally may be measured.

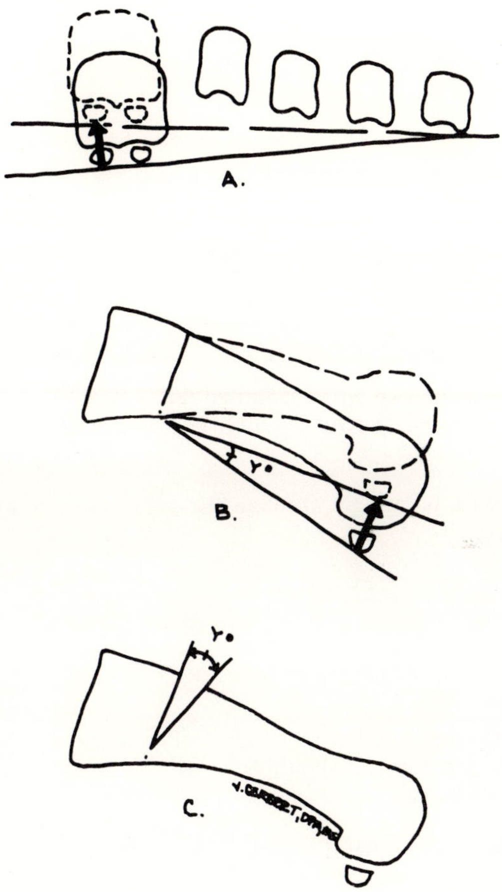

FIGURE 1
CALCULATION OF WEDGE TO BE REMOVED

A. A wire loop is constructed and held by a hemostat. It is placed in the center of the osteotomy.

B. The wires on each side of the osteotomy are passed so that they are placed through the loop.

C. The loop with the two wires is pulled dorsally through the center of the osteotomy. The loop is removed and the wires separated.

D. The distal wire is brought through the proximal wire and then both are twisted together.

E. One pulls the proximal wire (arrow) so that the distal wire is brought through the osteotomy. It should be noted that the pull is proximal toward the more stable site.

F. One can see that the distal wire may be tied to fix the osteotomy site.

G. This is a demonstration of the wire holding the bones in place after the osteotomy site has been closed.

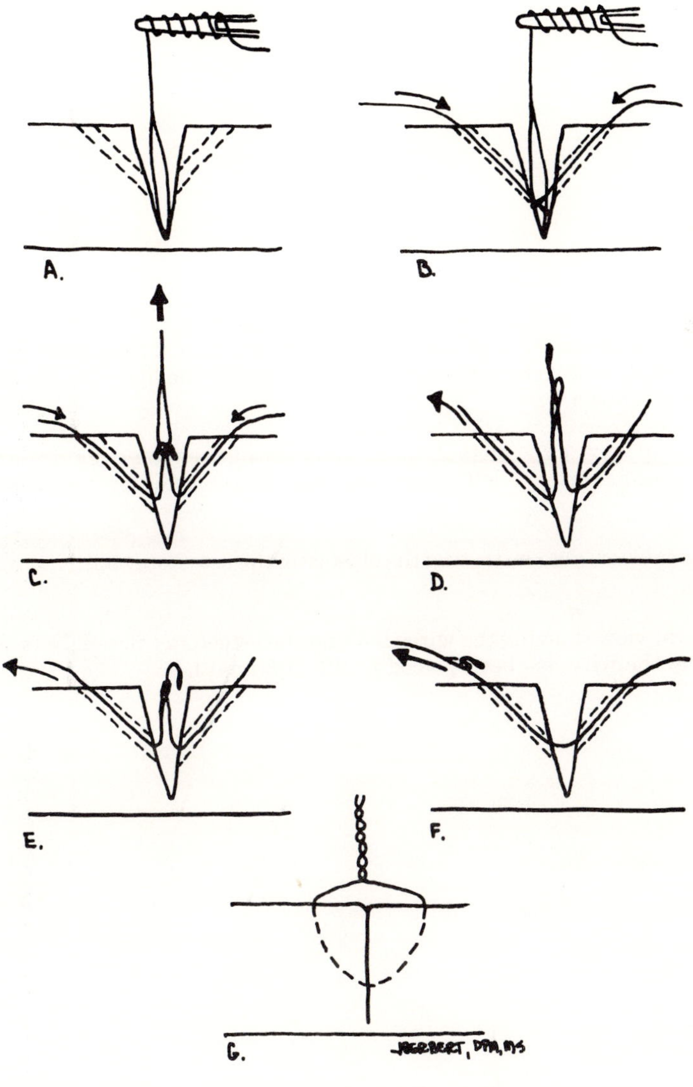

FIGURE 2
WIRE PASSING TECHNIQUE

A. This is a dorsal view of the first metatarsal. The shaded portion is the amount of bone to be removed. The placement of the holes for the fixation wires is shown.

B. A lateral view of the metatarsal demonstrating the wedge that is removed. The plantar cortex is left intact. The angle of the holes for wire fixation is noted.

C. A dorsal view demonstrating the closure of the osteotomy with the wires in place.

D. Lateral view showing the wires holding the osteotomy closed. Note the cut end of the wire has been placed in the proximal hole.

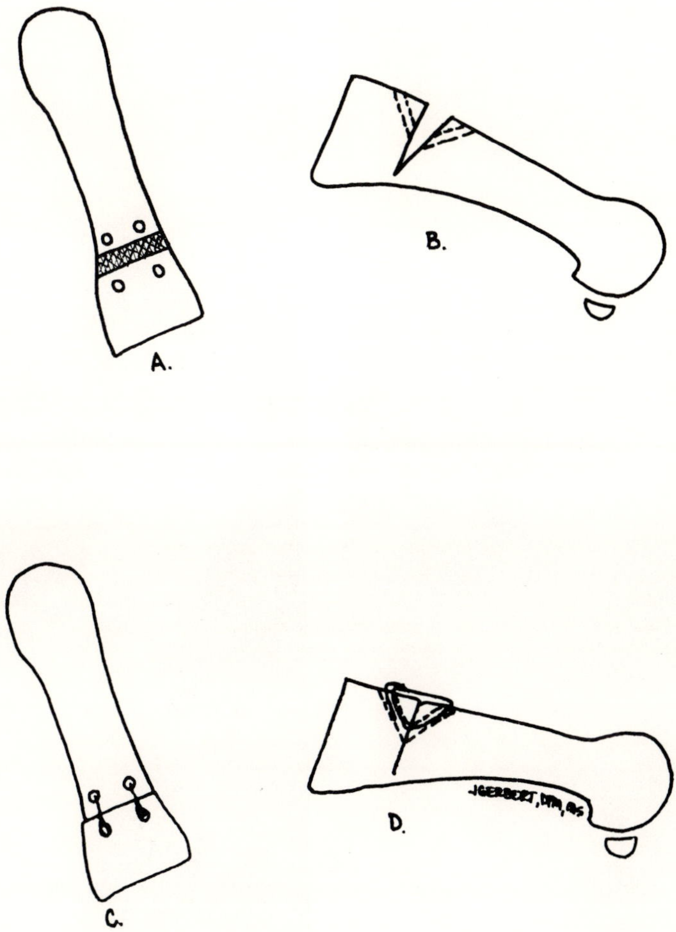

FIGURE 3
DORSAL WEDGE OSTEOTOMY

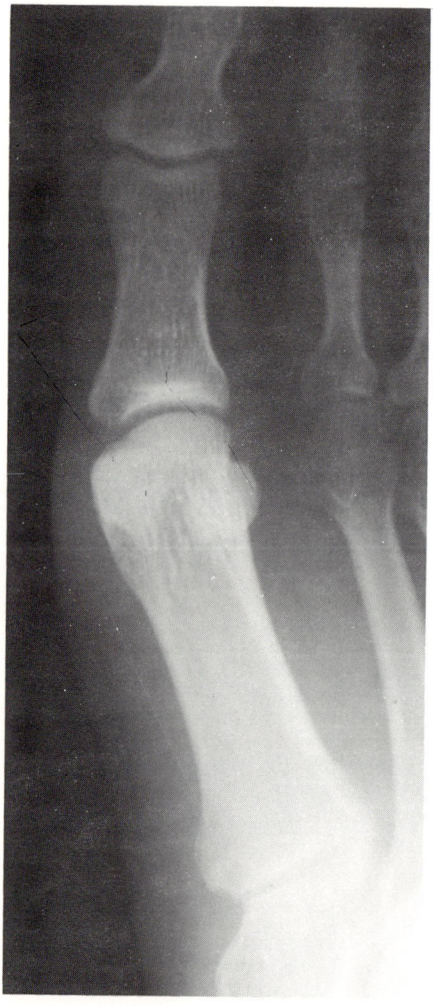

FIGURE 4A
PREOPERATIVE AP VIEW

Note the sesamoids appear normal in shape. The patient presented clinically with an intractable plantar keratoma under the first metatarsal.

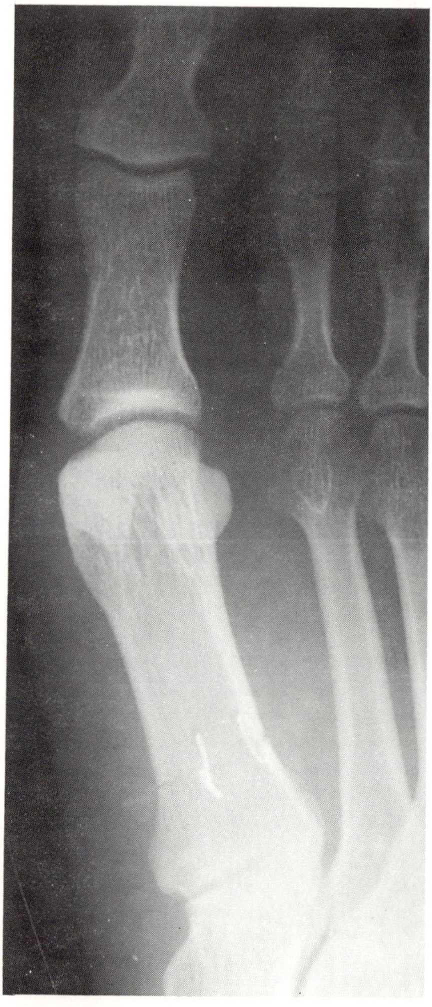

FIGURE 4B
POSTOPERATIVE AP VIEW

Note the location of the osteotomy in the proximal aspect of the metatarsal. The osteotomy was fixed with 2-0 monofilament steel.

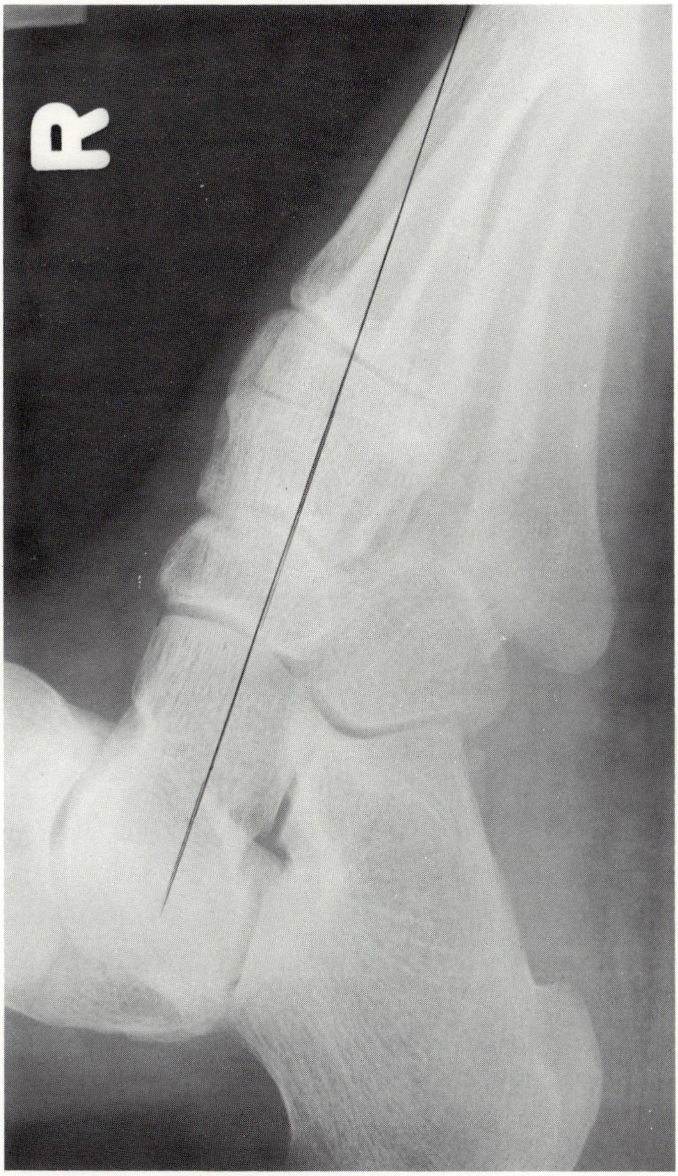

FIGURE 5A
PREOPERATIVE LATERAL VIEW

Note that the bisection of the talus passes dorsal to the head of the first metatarsal.

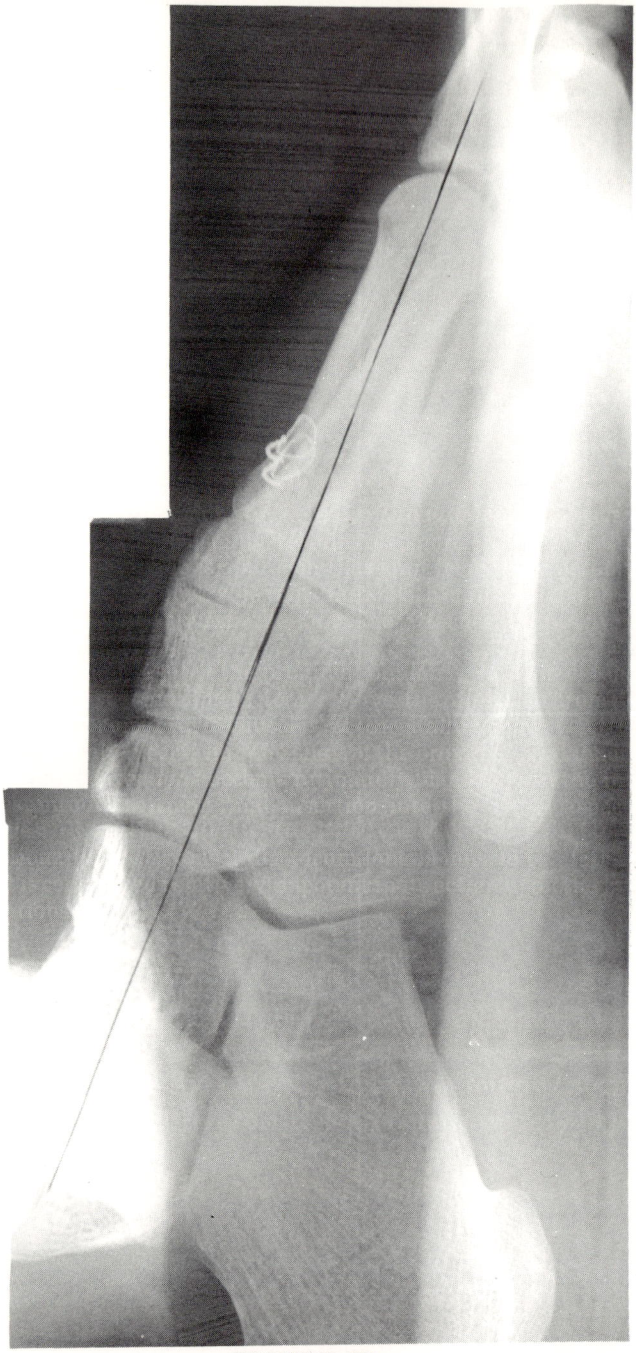

FIGURE 5B
POSTOPERATIVE LATERAL VIEW

Note the bisection of the talus passes through the first metatarsal head. This demonstrates the height that the first metatarsal has been raised.

4. Bi-Plane Wedge Osteotomy

This procedure utilizes the criteria previously described in the first monograph on Hallux abducto-valgus wedge osteotomy and a dorsal wedge osteotomy previously described in this monograph. The purpose is to reduce an increased metatarsus primus adductus angle and a plantar-flexed first ray.

Preoperative Signs

1. Hallux abducto valgus with bunion deformity may be present.
2. Bursa over the medial aspect of the first metatarsal head may be present.
3. Clinically, a metatarsus primus adductus is present.
4. Similar signs to soft tissue or arthroplasty procedures of the first metatarsal phalangeal joint.
5. Intractable plantar keratoma is present under the metatarsal head.
6. Atrophy of the plantar fat pad may be present.
7. A hallux hammertoe may be present.
8. A plantar flexed first ray may be present.
9. The tibial sesamoid is not prominent upon direct palpation.
10. The first metatarsal, when palpated with the foot loaded, is lower than the second metatarsal.
11. A rigid first ray is present.

Preoperative Symptoms

1. Pain with pressure on bunion deformity may be present.
2. Pain when wearing various types of foot gear may be present.
3. Pressure of the hallux against adjacent toes may be present.
4. Similar symptoms to soft tissue or arthroplasty procedures of the first metatarsal-phalangeal joint.
5. Pain plantar aspect of the first metatarsal head with or without foot gear.
6. Pain with direct pressure to the keratoma.
7. Inability to wear certain types of foot gear.
8. Pain exaggerated when wearing high-heeled foot gear.

Biomechanical Evaluation

1. Plantar flexed first ray is usually present.
2. Total forefoot valgus may be present.
3. The procedure may be performed with uncontrollable pronatory forces depending on the procedure at the first metatarsal-phalangeal joint.
4. Postoperative orthotic control should be utilized.

Preoperative X-ray Evaluation

1. Adequate bone density of the first metatarsal must be present.
2. Closure of the epiphysis of the first metatarsal should be present.
3. Metatarsus primus adductus angle must be greater than 12° in a rectus foot and 10° in an adductus foot.
4. First metatarsal should not be unduly short on X-ray.
5. Proximal articular set angle of less than 12° unless the metatarsal head is to be remodeled or a double osteotomy procedure performed.
6. Normal tibial sesamoid is present.
7. First metatarsal is depressed in relation to the second metatarsal.
8. A hallux abducto-valgus is usually present.

Surgical Procedure

An attempt to preoperatively calculate the amount of wedge to be taken should be made, although with this procedure it is difficult. A dorsal linear incision is made medial to the extensor hallucis longus tendon from the proximal phalanx of the hallux to the medial cuneiform. The indicated procedure is first performed at the metatarsal-phalangeal joint. Thus, when the osteotomy is completed and fixation obtained, the incisions need only to be sutured so as not to disturb the osteotomy site. The incision over the shaft of the metatarsal is deepened by sharp dissection. The extensor tendon is mobilized and is retracted laterally. A dorsal incision is made through the periosteum of the first metatarsal and is sharply dissected from the bone with a periosteal elevator. Seeburger retractors are placed in the wound to protect all soft tissue structures. With an oscillating hand piece on the power equipment the osteotomy is begun. It must be realized that the plantar medial aspect of the first metatarsal will be the only intact portion of bone remaining. The first cut is made across the metatarsal and perpendicular to the shaft, leaving the plantar cortex intact. The remainder of the osteotomy is then completed by taking portions of the bone from the proximal segment. The bone is resected from the dorsal aspect of the entire metatarsal so that it may be dorsiflexed and also from the lateral portion to allow for the adductory component of movement. It is necessary to completely transect the plantar portion of the bone except for the aforementioned plantar medial cortex. This will allow the distal portion of the metatarsal to be moved dorsal and lateral. Fixation is similar to that described for a dorsal wedge osteotomy of the first metatarsal. The periosteum is closed with 3-0 absorbable suture. The remainder of the incision is then closed at the metatarsal-phalangeal joint. The subcutaneous tissue is closed with 4-0 absorbable sutures. The skin is closed with 5-0 simple interrupted non-absorbable sutures.

Postoperative Management

The patient is placed in a short leg walking cast and allowed to ambulate in 24 to 48 hours when the cast dries. The patient is then seen weekly to check the cast and to make sure that there are no signs of infection. The cast is removed at the end of three weeks. The sutures are removed at this time and a postoperative X-ray is taken. The short leg walking cast is reapplied and left in place for another three weeks. At the end of this time the cast is removed and further X-rays are obtained. The osteotomy is usually healed enough to begin ambulation without plaster at this time. Bevin shoes and Ace bandages are given to the patient for one to two weeks to reduce post-cast edema. The patient should have negative impressions taken and orthotics constructed. The patient is usually able to return to normal foot gear in approximately eight weeks.

Advantages

1. The procedure reduces an osseous deformity in two planes.
2. The relationship of the first metatarsal to the second metatarsal may be determined during surgery.
3. The ability to control the amount of movement of the metatarsal during surgery.
4. The procedure may be combined with a procedure at the metatarsal-phalangeal joint.
5. The first metatarsal may be shortened if excessively long.
6. The ability to calculate preoperatively the amount of bone needed to be excised to achieve the desired correction.

Disadvantages

1. Longer healing phase due to osteotomy.
2. Internal fixation is necessary.
3. Prolonged disability and inconvenience for the patient is required.
4. Distraction of the osteotomy is possible which could result in poor alignment of the metatarsal.
5. Extremely small portion of bone left intact to act as a hinge.
6. Osteoporosis may ensue.
7. Possible complications from power equipment may occur.

A. The shaded area demonstrates the angle that the wedge needs to be removed. The area to be removed is greater on the lateral side to allow the metatarsal to be abducted. The holes that will be used for the wire fixation are shown.

B. The dotted area is the raw bone surfaces on the inner portion of the osteotomy. Note that the plantar medial cortex is the remaining hinge of bone.

C. The movement of the metatarsal in a lateral and dorsal direction is demonstrated. The metatarsal is shortened to a certain extent. The wire fixation is similar to that of a dorsal wedge osteotomy of the first metatarsal.

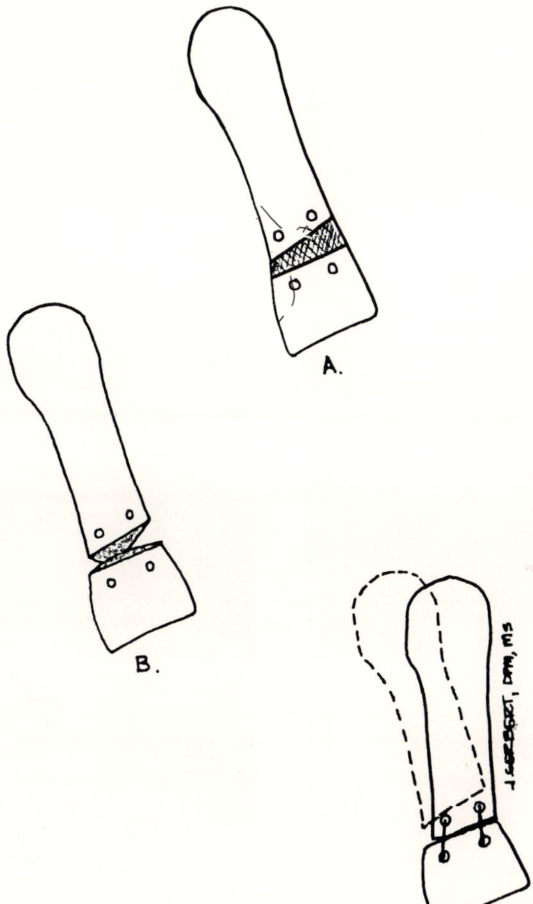

FIGURE 1
BI-PLANE WEDGE OSTEOTOMY

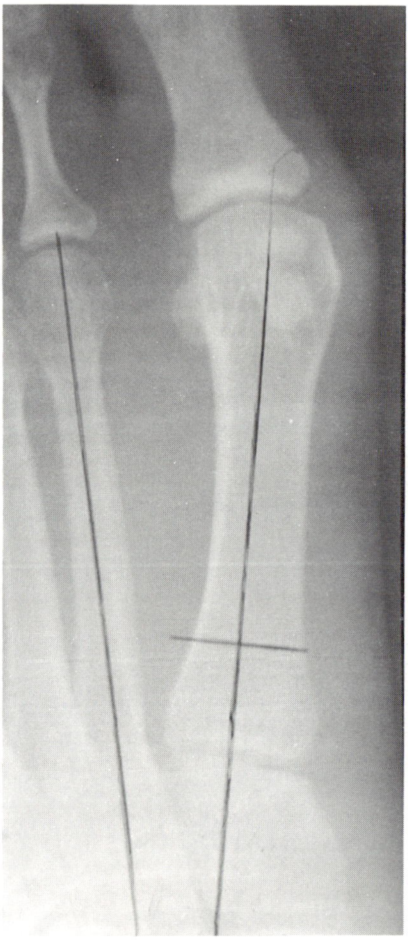

FIGURE 2A
PREOPERATIVE A-P X-RAY

This is an A-P preoperative view showing an increased metatarsus primus adductus angle of 13°. The first metatarso-phalangeal joint is in a deviated position. The line across the proximal portion of bone is at the approximate site of the osteotomy.

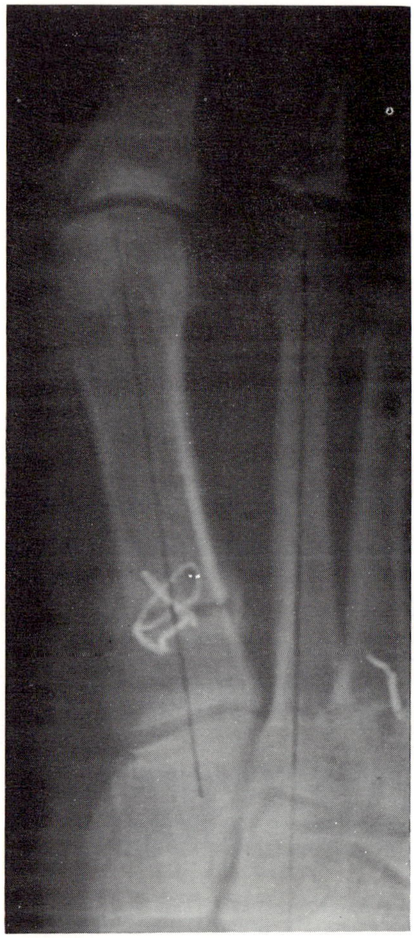

FIGURE 2B
POSTOPERATIVE A-P X-RAY

This is an A-P six week postoperative film showing a decrease in the metatarsus primus adductus angle to 9°. The wires that are shown in the first metatarsal have been crossed instead of being parallel with each other. Callus tissue may be seen surrounding the osteotomy site. The deviation of the first metatarso-phalangeal joint was also corrected.

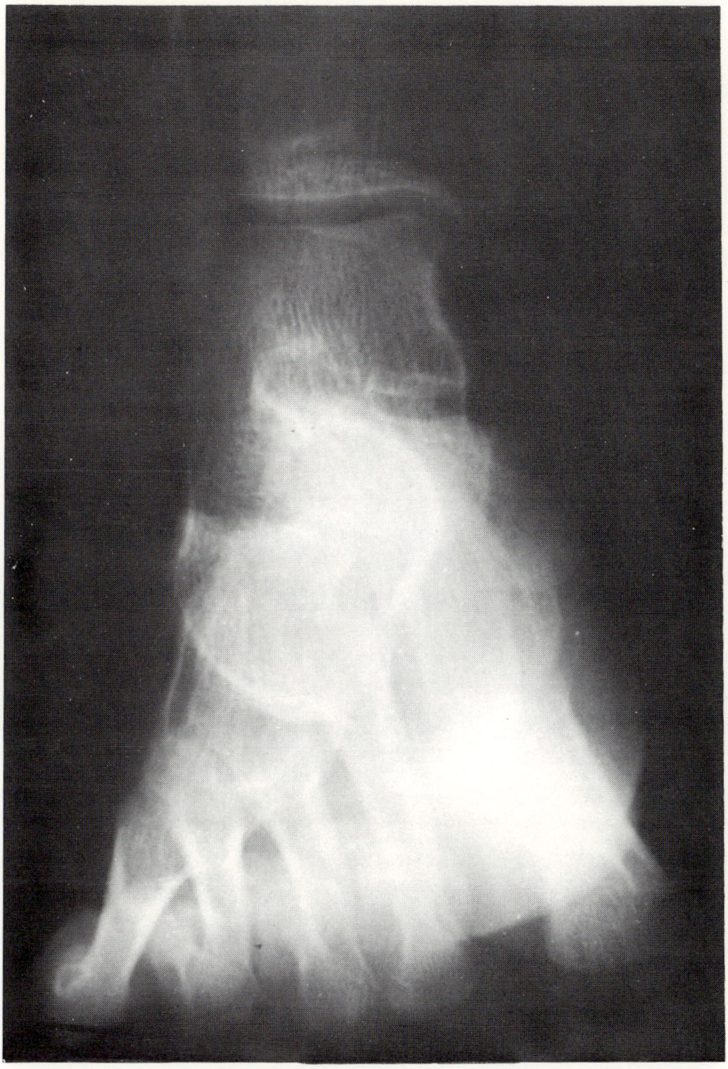

FIGURE 3A
PREOPERATIVE AXIAL X-RAY

An axial view of the foot shows that the first metatarsal is plantarflexed in relation to the other metatarsals. This is not an abnormal finding by itself. In the normal axial view, the first metatarsal is the most plantar, then the fifth metatarsal, fourth metatarsal, third metatarsal and, finally, second metatarsal.

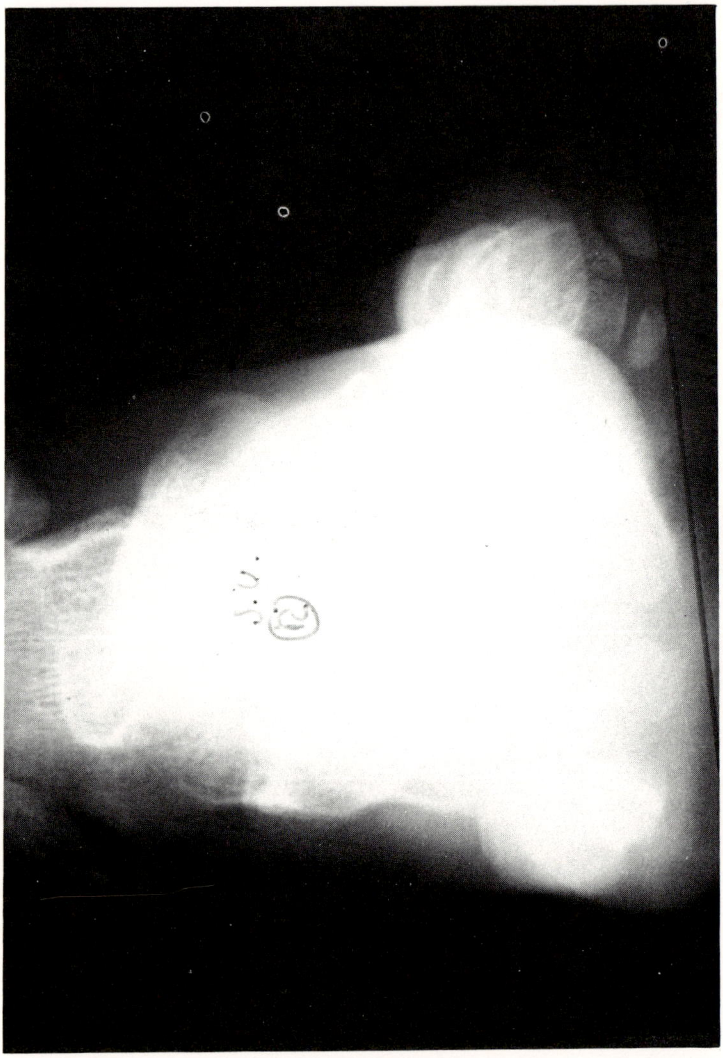

FIGURE 3B
POSTOPERATIVE AXIAL X-RAY

This is a six week postoperative axial view showing that the first metatarsal has been elevated. The first metatarsal is now on the same level as the second, while the third metatarsal appears depressed.

5. Crescentic Osteotomy

The use of the crescentic osteotomy for sub first metatarsal Intractable Plantar Keratomas (IPK) is not a commonly employed procedure. Quite often, the procedure is employed to reduce both a Primus Adductus and a Plantarflexed 1st Ray.

Preoperative Signs

1. An intractable plantar keratoma is present under the first metatarsal head.
2. The lesion is usually a nucleated shearing or fibrous nucleated shearing callous type.
3. The first metatarsal is in a plantar flexed position.
4. The dorsal excursion of the first metatarsal does not raise it above the level of the second metatarsal.

Preoperative Symptoms

1. Pain on direct palpation of the lesion.
2. The patient complains of plantar pain both in and out of shoes.
3. No pain on range of motion.

Biomechanical Evaluation

1. There is usually a varus rearfoot with no eversion beyond the vertical of the calcaneus.
2. Equinus deformity is an inconstant finding.
3. There may be either a plantar flexed first ray or a total forefoot valgus.
4. Dorsal excursion of the first ray does not go above the level of the second metatarsal.

Preoperative X-ray Evaluation

The preoperative X-ray findings are consistent with those discussed under Dorsal Wedge Osteotomy of the first metatarsal with the following exceptions:

1. Crescentic Osteotomy for Intractable Plantar Keratomas should be considered in those cases that show a relatively short first Metatarsal.
2. Cases done in conjunction with first metatarso-phalangeal joint arthroplasty in which dorsal jamming may occur post Dorsal Wedge Osteotomy.

Surgical Procedure

If the procedure is being performed in conjunction with a first metatarso-phalangeal joint arthroplasty, then a 6.5 cm. curvilinear skin incision is made from the middle of the proximal phalanx, to the metatarso-cuneiform joint. It is also possible to perform this procedure through two separate skin incisions. One for the first MPJ; the other for the base osteotomy. The choice of a one or two incision approach rests with the surgeon and is dependent upon the length of the first metatarsal (i.e., the shorter the metatarsal, the more the indication for one incision).

Attention is then directed to exposing the base area of the first metatarsal. The subcutaneous tissue is dissected freely since there are usually no vital structures encountered.

Immediately beneath the subcutaneous tissue lies the tendon of the Extensor Hallucis Longus. This structure must be preserved in its sheath to ensure success of the osteotomy.

Further dissection is necessary to expose the medial, lateral, and plantar aspect of the first metatarsal approximately 1 cm. from the base. Care must be exercised in lateral dissection to preserve the deep plantar perforating artery.

Dissection of the periosteum was once advocated as an essential part of the procedure. However, recent work has been done that shows this to be unnecessary.

A crescentic or curved cut is made in the bone, either with a power drill, or a crescentic blade of an oscillating saw. Use of the drill necessitates multiple drill holes and in effect removes approximately 2-3 millimeters of bone. By far, the best instrument is the crescentic blade attached to the oscillating saw. Here, a clean cut is made that reflects the width of the blade and does not appreciably shorten bone.

In a combined procedure that corrects both the Primus Adductus and Plantarflexed First Ray, the cut is made from medial to lateral beginning dorsally.

When employing this procedure solely for the correction of a Plantarflexed First Ray, the cut can be made from dorsal to plantar approaching from the medial side.

The cut is made completely through the bone in either approach and the metatarsal is moved to its new position.

Since complete transection is made, internal wire sutures should not be employed. Rather, external Kirschner wire fixation is utilized.

The amount of correction necessary will determine whether one or two K-wires are necessary. The K-wire should be introduced from distal to proximal, starting away from the osteotomy and angling through the proximal portion of bone into the cuneiform area.

Closure is then accomplished in layers utilizing 4-0 chromic or Dexon suture material. Skin closure is left to the choice of the surgeon.

The K-wire is cut either beneath the skin or protruding about 0.5 cm. from the point of entry. The wound and wire is covered with a non-adherent dressing and well padded with bandage.

A below-knee cast is then applied. Position of the metatarsal is the direct responsibility of the surgeon and is the most important part of the procedure.

Postoperative Management

The patient is casted in a short leg walking cast for 6-8 weeks with ambulation commencing 3-4 days postoperative. Cast change is done at the 3rd or 4th postoperative week with K-wire and suture removal and recasting being performed. X-rays are taken 6 weeks postoperative to determine the extent of healing. If it is sufficient the cast is removed, an ace bandage or flexible cast is applied and a postoperative shoe is dispensed. The patient is instructed to ambulate with limits.

Postoperative edema, one of the most persistent problems post-osteotomy, is controlled by elevation, ace wraps, or supportive stockings. Return to shoes is dictated by the patients postoperative appearance, usually about 10-12 weeks postoperatively.

Advantage

1. Preserves length of bone.

Disadvantage

1. Must be held with K wires.
2. Difficult to relocate in desired position calculated preoperatively.

This represents a diagramatic presentation of a first metatarsal crescentic osteotomy. This procedure can be used to dorsally locate the first metatarsal, but is more often used for metatarsus primus adductus. Fixation is accomplished via Kirschner Wires.

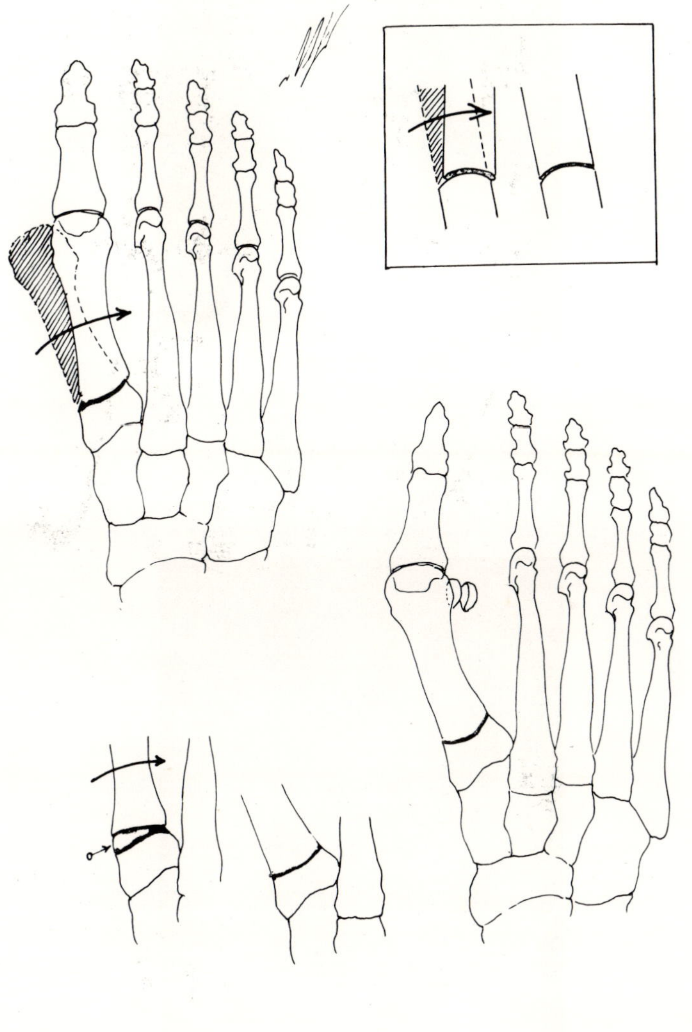

FIGURE 1
CRESCENTIC OSTEOTOMY

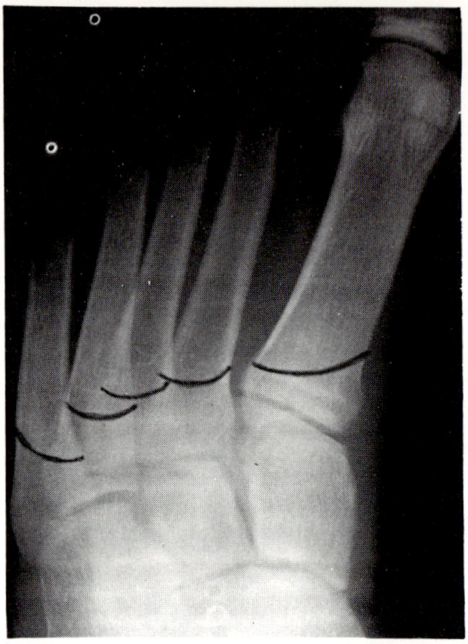

FIGURE 2A
PREOPERATIVE X-RAY

Preoperative determination for crescentic osteotomies to be performed at the bases of the metatarsals.

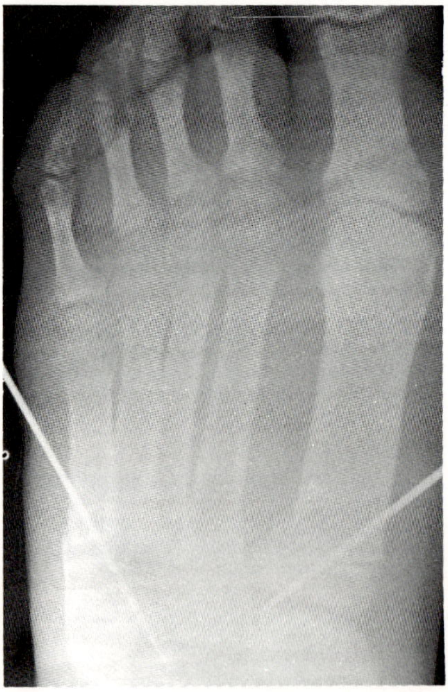

FIGURE 2B
POSTOPERATIVE X-RAY

K-wiring of the metatarsals.

6. Sir Robert Jones Procedure

This procedure is a transposition of the extensor hallucis longus tendon to the head of the first metatarsal. A fusion of the interphalangeal joint is usually performed in addition to the transposition. Kirk et al devised a ledge tenodesis of the extensor hallucis longus to avoid some of the problems with the Jones procedure.

Preoperative Signs

1. An intractable plantar keratoma under the first metatarsal.
2. Atrophy of the plantar fat pad may be present.
3. A hallux hammertoe is usually present.
4. A hallux abductus may be present.
5. A normal range of motion of the first metatarsal-phalangeal joint should be present.
6. The first metatarsal should have a range of motion to above the second metatarsal head.
7. The range of motion of the first metatarsal-phalangeal joint should not be painful.
8. Crepitus and/or pain may be present in the interphalangeal joint of the hallux.

Preoperative Symptoms

1. Pain plantar to the first metatarsal during ambulation with or without foot gear.
2. Pain with direct pressure to the plantar lesion.
3. Inability to wear certain types of shoes.
4. Pain over the interphalangeal joint of the hallux may be present.
5. Pain over the medial aspect of the first metatarsal head may be present.

Biomechanical Evaluation

1. A mobile plantarflexed first ray is present.
2. This procedure can be performed in the presence of uncontrollable pronatory forces.
3. A functional or accomodative orthotic is needed postoperatively.

Preoperative X-ray Evaluation

1. The first metatarsal is the lowest on the axial view.
2. The tibial sesamoid is normal in appearance.

3. The first metatarsal-phalangeal joint shows no degenerative changes.
4. A hallux hammertoe may be present.
5. Degenerative arthritis may be present in the interphalangeal joint of the hallux.

Surgical Procedure

Two semi-elliptical incisions are made over the interphalangeal joint of the hallux. The intervening skin is excised. The tendon is sectioned as far distally as possible, to allow entrance to the interphalangeal joint, and freed from its sheath. The collateral ligaments are incised so that the articular surfaces may be delivered into the wound. The oscillating blade of the microstryker is used to resect the articular surfaces of the interphalangeal joint. They are cut parallel to each other so that the hallux hammertoe may be reduced. An internal wire fixation may be used to fix the parts, which obviates the need for a Kirschner wire. A drill hole is made from the dorsal to the plantar surface of each phalanx 3mm. from the cut surfaces. Number 2-0 monofilament wire is doubled and passed through each hole. After retrieving each wire through the void the distal wire is pulled through the center of the proximal wire. The proximal wire then is pulled bringing the distal wire with it. After disengaging the two wires, the remaining wire is tightened to obtain compression of the raw surfaces. The subcutaneous tissue is closed over the wire with 3-0 or 4-0 absorbable suture and the skin is closed with 5-0 nonabsorbable suture.

A linear incision is made over the dorsum of the first metatarsal-phalangeal joint medial to the extensor hallucis longus tendon. The subcutaneous tissue is freed by sharp and blunt dissection to expose the capsule of the first metatarsal-phalangeal joint. The extensor hallucis longus tendon is identified and freed from its sheath and pulled through from the distal incision. If the capsule need not be entered, a drill hole is placed from medial to lateral just proximal to the capsule. If the first metatarsal must be exposed the capsule is incised with a dorsal linear incision. The head of the metatarsal is completely freed from the collateral ligaments so that it can be delivered into the wound. The prominent medial eminence is resected at this time and the drill hole completed. A suture is placed through the end of the tendon. The suture is then threaded through the hole and the tendon pulled through. The metatarsal is dorsiflexed to its intended level and the foot is placed in its loaded position. The tendon is brought dorsally and sutured to itself with 3-0 nonabsorbable suture. The capsule is closed if necessary with 3-0 absorbable suture; the subcutaneous tissue closed with 4-0 absorbable suture and skin is closed with 5-0 suture.

Postoperative Management

A dry compression bandage and a below the knee weight bearing cast is applied. This is to put the tendon at rest during the healing stage. The cast is left in place for two to three weeks and removed at the end of this period to remove sutures. X-rays are taken at this time. The patient is put back into a plaster cast for another two to three weeks. When this cast is removed a postoperative wooden shoe is utilized for one to two weeks. The patient can get back to regular shoes at the end of this period of time. Orthotic therapy is begun at this time.

Advantages

1. The primary osseous deformity is reduced.
2. The range of motion of the first metatarsal-phalangeal joint is maintained.
3. The stability of the first metatarsal-phalangeal joint is maintained.
4. A hallux abductus deformity may be reduced.
5. The hallux hammertoe deformity is reduced.

Disadvantages

1. The extensor tendon may not hold the metatarsal in the corrected position.
2. The first metatarsal may be moved too high.
3. The range of motion of the first metatarsal may be decreased.
4. The arthrodesis site may rotate if a Kirschner wire is used.
5. Pseudoarthrosis of the interphalangeal joint.
6. Fracture of the arthrodesis site may occur.

A. This lateral diagram depicts a hallux hammertoe in conjunction with a plantarflexed first metatarsal. The retrograde force from the contracted hallux produces a plantarflexory action on the metatarsal.

B. Throughout the remaining diagrams, one must keep in mind that the interphalangeal fusion and the extensor hallucis longus transposition are actually two separate procedures. In this diagram, the extensor hallucis longus tendon is transected as far distally as possible. One is then able to enter the interphalangeal joint, resect the articular cartilage to create a fusion. Note the position of the hole in the first metatarsal for the transposition of the tendon.

C. A dorsal view showing the transection of the tendon and resection of bone. The dotted lines in the head of the first metatarsal represent the drill hole.

D. The interphalangeal joint is fixed with a through-and-through 2-0 monofilament stainless steel suture. This fixation affords excellent compression while not allowing rotation. An easy method for threading the suture through the hole is demonstrated in this diagram. A wire suture is folded in half and the blind end is fed through the hole from lateral. The suture is passed through the wire which is then pulled in the direction of the arrow. This in turn pulls the suture through the hole.

E. The through-and-through wire fixation of the interphalangeal joint is shown. Also one may note the tendon as it is directed through the metatarsal head.

F. A dorsal view depicts the compression at the fusion site. The tendon has been threaded through the hole and is brought dorsally into place where it is sutured upon itself.

G. Final fixation of the interphalangeal joint is noted. The metatarsal has been raised and held in this position by the tendon. The hallux hammertoe has been reduced. The proximal phalanx is now sitting in a much better relation compared with the head of the metatarsal.

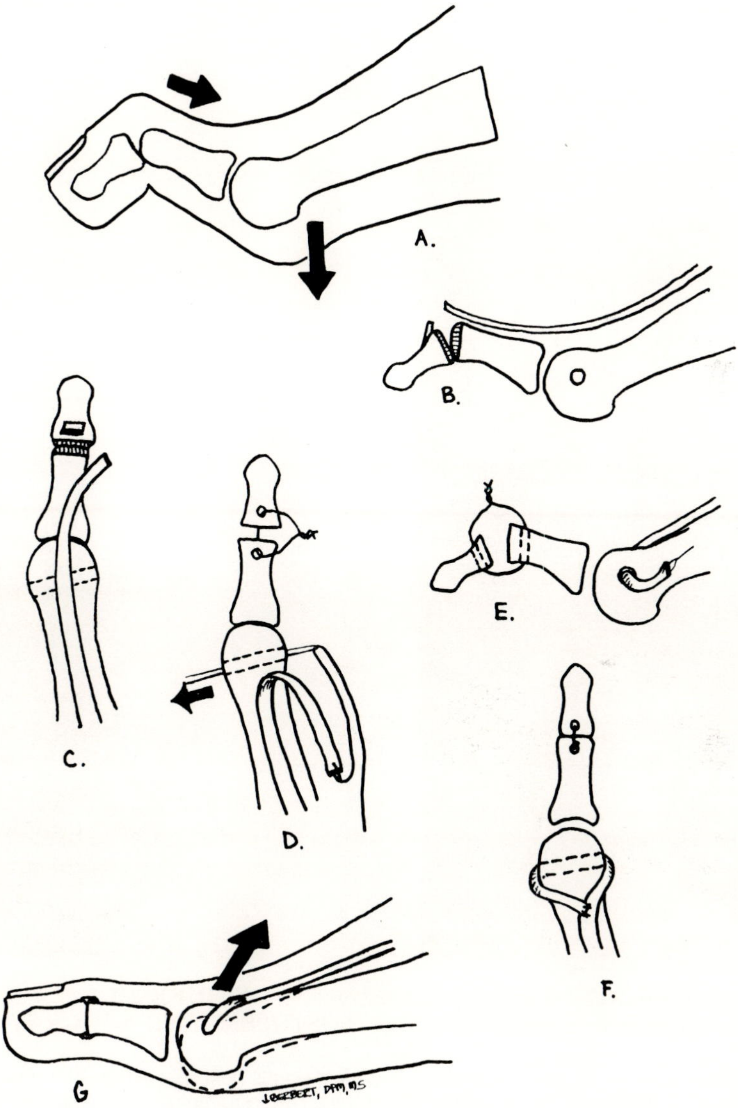

FIGURE 1
SIR ROBERT JONES PROCEDURE

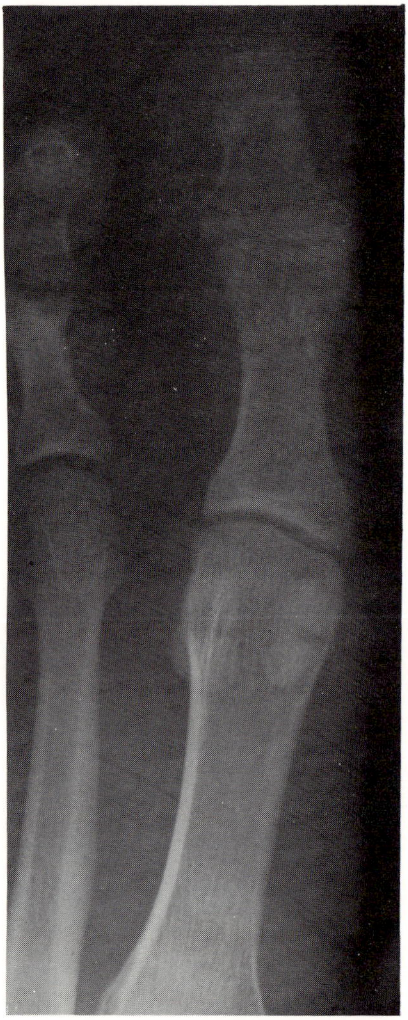

FIGURE 2A
PREOPERATIVE A-P X-RAY

A preoperative A-P view shows a contracted hallux at the interphalangeal joint. An increase in soft tissue density due to the contracture is noted medial to the interphalangeal joint. The metatarso-phalangeal joint space is minimally decreased due to the dorsal dislocation.

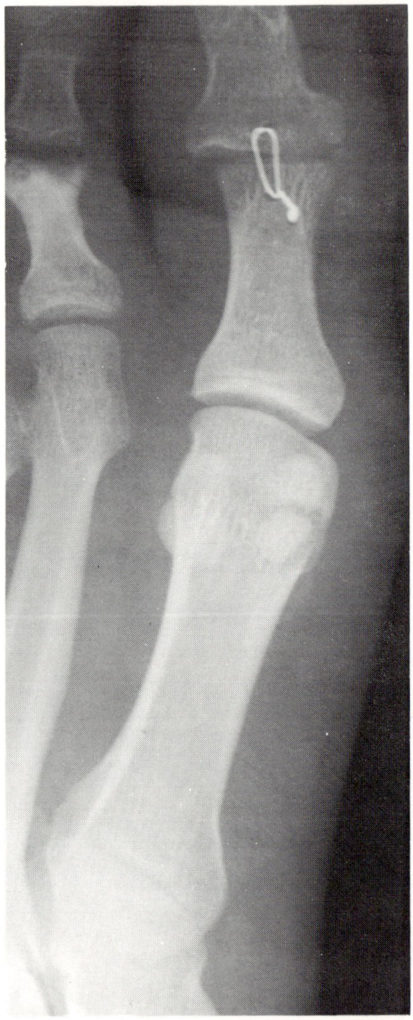

FIGURE 2B
POSTOPERATIVE A-P X-RAY

A two week postoperative A-P X-ray shows that the articular surfaces of the interphalangeal joint have been resected. A steel suture is being used to maintain the ends in contact. One may note that the hole for the tendon transposition is passing through the sesamoidal area. The metatarso-phalangeal joint space is increased due to reduction of the dislocation.

Bibliography

DuVries, H. L.: *Surgery of the Foot,* Ed. Inman, V.; 3rd Edition. St. Louis, C. V. Mosby Co., 1973, pp. 535.

Giannestras, N. J.: *Foot Disorders; Medical and Surgical Management,* Philadelphia, Lea & Febiger, 1973, pp. 319.

Jones, R.: *Notes on Military Orthopaedics,* New York, P. B. Hoebber, 1917, pp. 38-57.

Jones, R.: The soldier's foot and the treatment of common deformities of the foot. Part II: Claw-Foot. *Brit. Med. Journal,* **1**:749-753, 1916.

Kirk, A. A., Dunkle, H. M. and Waine, H. J.: Ledge tenodesis of the extensor hallucis longus: A substitution for the jones operation. *J. Bone & Joint Sur.,* **53-A**:774-776, June 1971.

B. Second, Third and Fourth Metatarsal IPK

The following illustrations (Figures 1, 2, and 3) represent some basic considerations which the surgeon should keep in mind concerning the lesser metatarsals before contemplating osteotomy procedures to shorten a bone, creating a different metatarsal parabola.

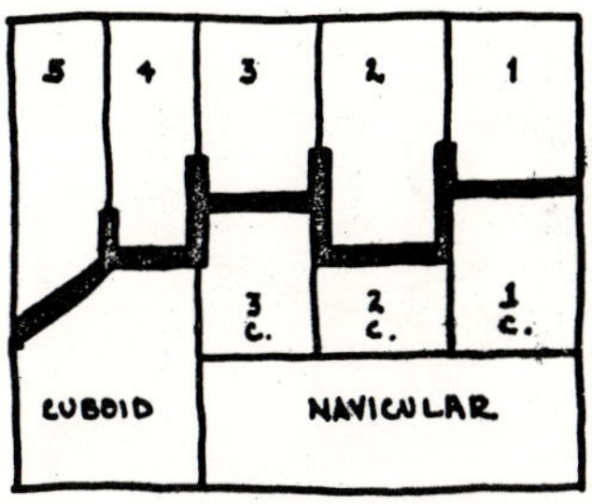

FIGURE 1

Schematic drawing showing approximate level of bases of metatarsals with respect to each other and their proximal bones.

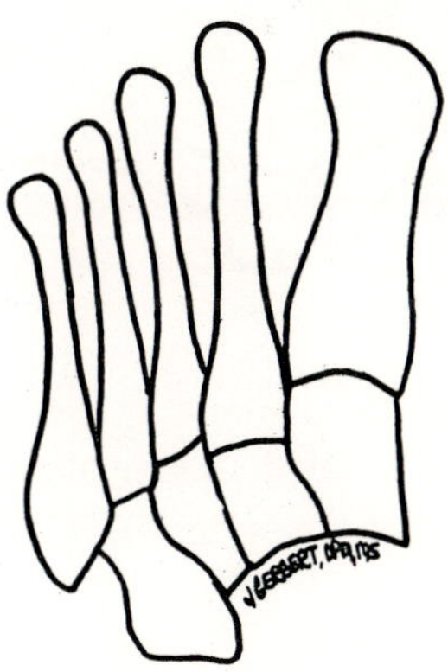

FIGURE 2

Drawing of actual structure of the five metatarsals and their relation to each other.

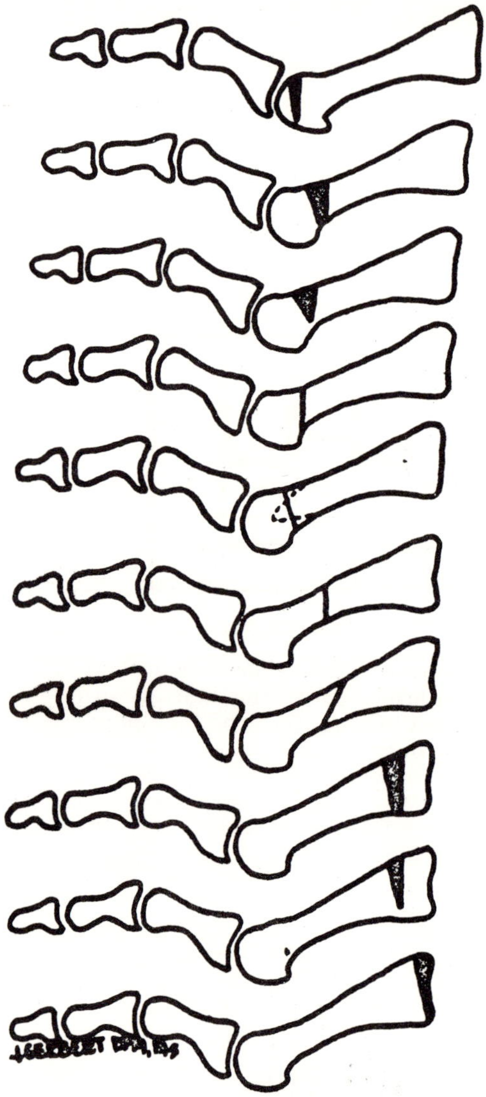

FIGURE 3

Different types of osteotomies to elevate lesser Metatarsals.

1. Dorsal Metatarsal Osteotomy

The procedure to be discussed in this chapter was first performed at the California Podiatry Hospital in 1965. Osteotomies for the treatment of intractable plantar keratomas have been performed for many years. Procedures have been described to osteotomize metatarsals at the base, at the mid-shaft, at the neck, and at the head. The relative ease of performing this procedure in cancellous bone has proven to be very successful. The problems of osteotomy surgery are that the patient and the doctor are not in line for the same result, so that a success in the doctor's mind, is not always a success in the patient's mind. It is important to ascertain whether the patient is concerned with the pain alone, or the pain and the lesion together. This simply means that if the patient desires not only the freedom of pain from the plantar lesion but also the complete eradication of the lesion, then the surgeon must see to it that the plantar lesion is either excised, so as to afford the cosmetic relief of the condition, or assured in his own mind that the procedure will result in the dissolution of the lesion. This probably is a number one problem in surgical procedures for plantar lesions. Throughout the history we have seen why partial osteotomies have not been successful. The lesion basically, has been treated as a cause and effect-type lesion, whereas it is really a structure, causing enough shear against the plantar skin to create the mechanical lesion.

The performing of a dorsal wedge osteotomy is really realigning structure so that the etiology can be changed and therefore the lesion would be resolved, along with its symptoms. It is not unusual to have to realign multiple metatarsals in order to accomplish a desired result. Transfer lesions will be avoided by acknowledging the fact that more than one metatarsal contributes to the symptoms being presented.

Preoperative Signs

1. Isolated hyperkeratotic lesions under the lesser metatarsal head area.
2. Confluent hyperkeratotic lesions involving more than one metatarsal area.
3. An adventitious bursitis under a metatarsal head or under multiple metatarsal heads.
4. An atrophy under plantar fat pad under the metatarsal head area.
5. A forefoot equinus deformity.
6. A forefoot varus deformity.
7. A forefoot valgus deformity.

8. A sub-talar varus with a compensated mid-tarsal joint.
9. A sub-talar varus with an un-compensated mid-tarsal joint.
10. A sub-talar valgus with a compensated mid-tarsal joint.
11. A sub-talar valgus with an un-compensated mid-tarsal joint.
12. An equinus deformity at the ankle joint, either osseous or soft tissue.

Preoperative Symptoms

1. A plantar hyperkeratotic lesion located under one or more metatarsal head areas, which has not responded to conservative treatment.
2. Pain in the hyperkeratotic lesion.
3. Burning or paraesthesias in the plantar lesion.
4. Swelling around the plantar lesion.
5. Thick plantar skin which the patient objects to.

Biomechanical Evaluation

1. The possible existence of an equinus deformity in the rear foot.
2. A sub-talar varus with or without a compensated mid-tarsal joint.
3. A sub-talar valgus with or without a compensated mid-tarsal joint.
4. A forefoot varus with or without compensated sub-talar joint.
5. A forefoot valgus with or without a compensated sub-talar joint.

Preoperative X-ray Evaluation

1. Possible equinus changes in the rear foot.
   a) A decrease in the declination angle of the calcaneus.
   b) Plantar flexion and forward displacement of the talus on the calcaneus.
   c) Jamming of the neck of the talus into the navicular.
   d) Increase in density of the posterior facet of the navicular.
   e) Possible hypertrophy of the head and neck area of the talus.
   f) Plantar flexion of one or more metatarsals on an axial view.
   g) Hypertrophy of the plantar aspect of the metatarsal.
   h) Arthritic changes at the lesser metatarsal-phalangeal joint level; these may or may not be seen.

Surgical Procedure

The procedure can be performed as an in-patient or an out-patient in an office environment. The technique for performing the osteotomy as described in this section, will apply to both an in-patient and an out-patient type procedure. Approximately a six cm dorsal linear incision is initiated over the base of the metatarsal in question. The usual problem for the novice surgeon attempting this procedure is identifying the basal areas of the metatarsal in question. The best way in teaching this procedure is to always go lateral to the extensor tendon of the toe in question. This is even more accentuated in a patient who has a metatarsal adductus deformity. The incision is carried through the sub-cutaneous tissue and the sub-cutaneous venous structures. They should be clamped or ligated as necessary. The procedure may be performed under a pneumatic cuff or under a wet field. This is strictly the surgeon's choice. If, after the superficial fascia is incised, the surgeon does not find himself on the dorsal surface of the metatarsal, then he should discontinue sharp dissection and use blunt dissection until he isolates the structure. There is no need to disrupt the interosseous muscle belly, other than to free it from the surrounding periosteum of the metatarsal in question. The classic description of this procedure is that it is performed approximately 1 cm distal to the metatarsal cuneiform joint. The reason for this figure is that it is at approximately 1 cm that we run into cancellous bone and this is the area of choice, because of its relative vascularity which is excellent for good bony heeling. This 1 cm represents the area where the metatarsal starts to fan out. The surgeon should do his work at just about the level of the fanning of the metatarsal so that he may get adequate exposure of both sides of his osteotomy site. By use of a rotary burr, which can be used on a power-driven instrument, or an oscillating saw attached to a power saw, or even an osteotome and mallet, if that is the surgeon's choice, a section of bone is removed at the area 1 cm distal to the metatarsal cuneiform joint. The usual width of this wedge is approximately 2 to 3 mm in size. The wedge should be perpendicular to the sagittal long axis of the shaft. It is better to raise the metatarsal to the level of the adjacent metatarsals, rather than above, for this creates as much of a problem as a plantar-flex metatarsal, with transfer lesions being a complication. After the wedge of bone is removed, the plantar cortex is examined to make sure that it is intact. The wedge is an incomplete wedge so that the plantar cortex remains intact creating a green stick-type fracture, where in actuality, only one wall is insulted and we don't have to worry about lateral displacement of the osteotomy, nor do we have to worry about rotation of the osteotomy site. This is one of the distinct advantages of this procedure, if performed correctly. If a rotary instrument is used, it is recommended that a 2 mm femoral osteotomy burr be used. Three holes are then drilled on the dorsal aspect of the metatarsal; two holes may be drilled but a three hole closure will prevent any rotation. The hole actually comes out at the intermedullary area of the bone. Drill two holes distally to the osteotomy site and one proximally. Either 2-0 braided or 2-0 monofilament wire is then passed through the hole, respectively. The best technique for passing wire through the hole is using a small wire to form a loop which is passed through the hole to receive the single strand of wire passed through the proximal hole and then it is pulled out in total through the distal hole. After the wire is placed through both holes it is then grasped with a straight forceps and the assistant closes the osteotomy site, making sure that there is good surface to surface contact of the bone, and turns the instrument on itself until the wire becomes braided and the osteotomy site maintains its own integrity. The subject of compression always comes in at this time and, as we know, too much compression sometimes causes enough atrophy at the osteotomy site to loosen up and work against the end result. There should be just enough compression to maintain good bone to bone contact. The wire is then cut long enough so that the remaining piece of wire can be passed over the osteotomy site and into one of the holes distally, so that it does not offend any soft tissue surrounding it. At this point a flush of Saline solution should be performed to lavage the entire surgical area. Sub-cutaneous tissues are then closed with 3 or 4 chromic sutures or whatever the surgeon desires and then skin closure is performed, with the material of choice of the surgeon. Again, it must be reiterated that if the surgeon feels that there are two metatarsals causing the lesion, then both should be osteotomized at the same time; many times the two can be taken care of through the same incision and the same surgical approach. The postoperative management of the patient is of paramount importance. The dressing is put on so that a plantar buttress is applied under the metatarsal to prevent it from dropping, even at rest. A slipper cast, similar to the one applied for casting of orthotics, may be applied to the plantar aspect of the foot, to give plantar immobilization to the osteotomy site. Most often a simple dressing of sterile 4 by 4 and Kling and an elastic bandage on top of that, such as Coban, is sufficient. The patient is allowed to ambulate that day in a postoperative hard sole shoe. The postoperative course of events usually shows a mild amount of swelling around the osteotomy site. This is usually due to the fact that the patient is walking on a surgical fracture site and the area becomes swollen due to this insult, but it should not be regarded as a problem to manage, nor should it cause the patient to remain at bedrest.

For those surgeons doing osteotomy surgery for the first time, it should be stated that the decision to place the patient into a normal postoperative shoe without dressing, or to allow them to assume their normal work in normal shoes should not be based on the X-ray changes which are apparent. In most instances there can be resorption or a visible osteotomy line for up to 6 months. Upon clinical examination, one can find that there is no sign of pseudoarthroses, due to the fact that there is no motion clinically available or pain at the osteotomy site and one must assume that there is a good fibrous anklyosis and bony healing and pro-callus would be visible shortly.

There may be significant osteoporosis because the patient is not ambulating normally. Again the treatment for this should be to encourage ambulation so that normal stress will cause recalcification of the osteotomy and bones around the area.

Postoperative Management

As described under the surgical section, the management of the patient is that he is able to ambulate immediately after the surgical procedure is performed. He may or may not be put into a slipper type cast. It is not necessary to place these patients into a short-leg cast, unless the procedure is performed for such things as metatarsus adductus with plantar lesions under all four or five metatarsals. Most patients require no more than mild analgesics to maintain pain. All patients are casted for orthotics on the first redressing so that the cause of the original problem and the mechanical problems within the foot and leg may be controlled to afford a maximum postoperative effort to avoid further lesions. The patient usually has the sutures removed within 10 to 14 days.

Advantages

1. Ease of performing the surgical technique.
2. Minimal worry about where the metatarsal will be situated after surgery.
3. Minimal displacement concern in either the sagittal axis or the transverse axis and no concern about rotation.
4. Good healing tendency.
5. No extensive disability due to procedure.

Disadvantages

1. Internal fixation by use of wire is required.
2. The operative technique is slightly more involved than with simpler procedures, such as plantar condylectomoies and osteoclasis procedures, but the advantages far outweigh the disadvantages.

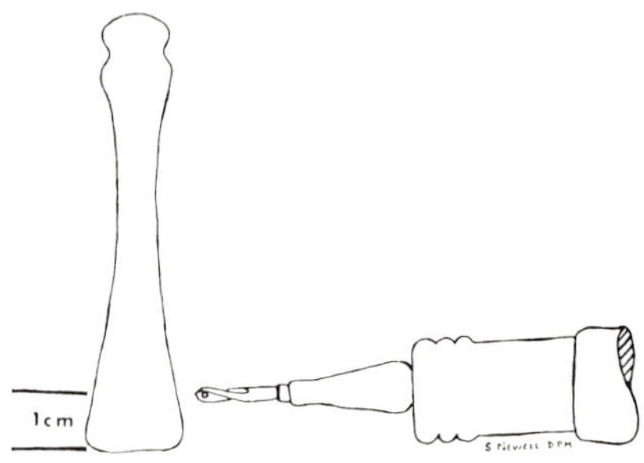

FIGURE 4
DORSAL WEDGE OSTEOTOMY

Osteotomy site level is approximately 1cm. from joint or at the level where the base and shaft join. Clearance of adjacent metatarsals is required.

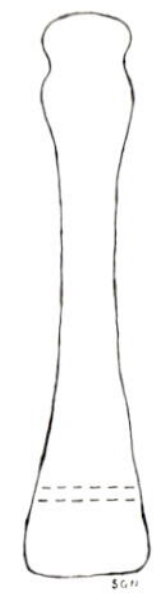

FIGURE 5
WEDGE WIDTH SCORE

Approximately 2mm. wide perpendicular to sagittal long axis of shaft. We have found 2mm is sufficient in almost all lesser metatarsal osteotomies and, many times, too large.

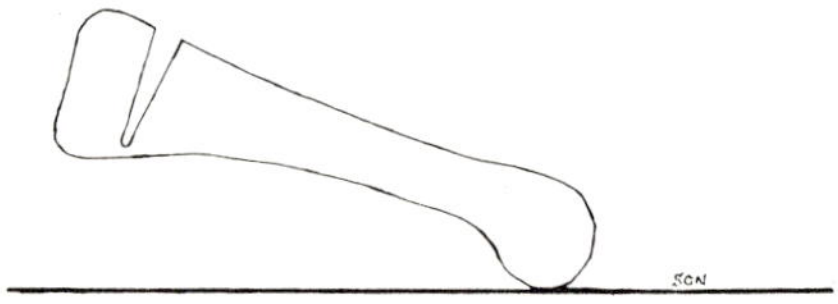

FIGURE 6
WEDGE REMOVED

The bone is cut down to, but not through, the plantar cortex, with the widest point of wedge being 2mm.

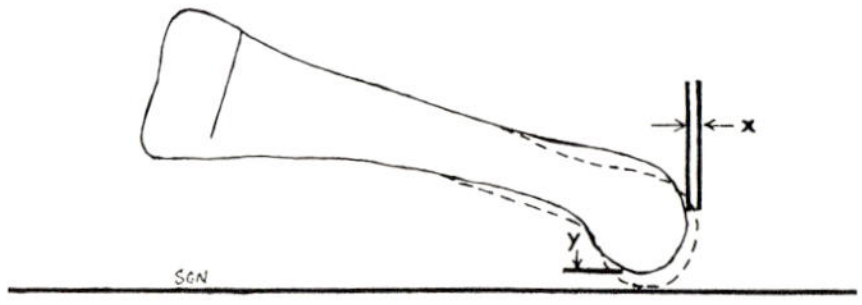

FIGURE 7
CLOSING OF WEDGE

When the distal segment is mobilized dorsally to close the wedge, the plantar cortex should be thin enough to bend. Closure of osteotomy site raises metatarsal (y) and slightly shortens metatarsal (x). This is advantageous as the intrinsic muscles will be slightly relaxed, which they can absorb. If a wedge is added, the intrinsic structures are placed on a stretch and can undergo contractural changes.

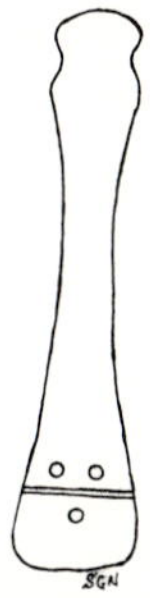

FIGURE 8
THREE HOLE FIXATION

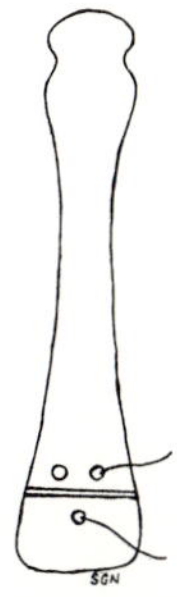

FIGURE 9
WIRING

Two strands of 00 braided stainless steel sutures are placed from the proximal stump hole, one each to the distal holes.

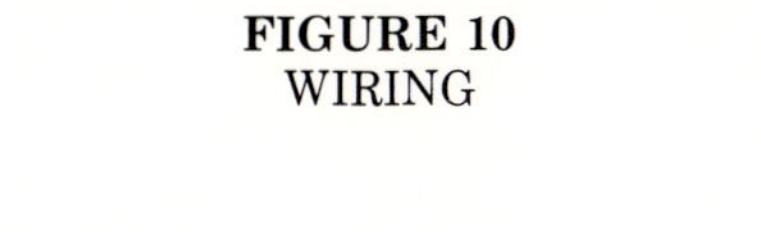

FIGURE 10
WIRING

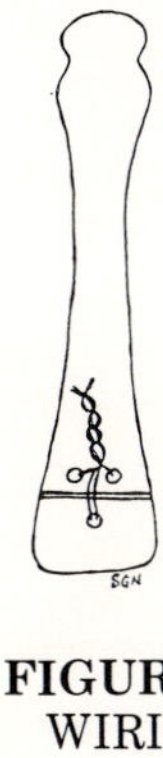

FIGURE 11
WIRING

The strands are then rotated from top to produce the desired compression. If the wedge is too large, the wound is left gaping as long as the plantar cortex is intact. The metatarsal should be elevated just to the level desired.

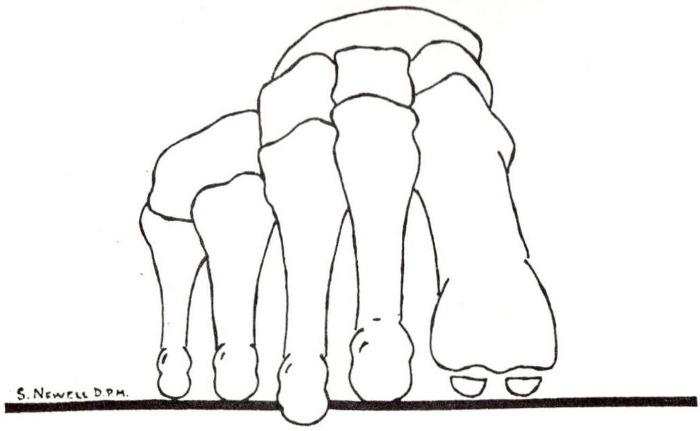

FIGURE 12
PLANTARLY DECLINED
LESSER METATARSAL

Foot is fully loaded in position of function.

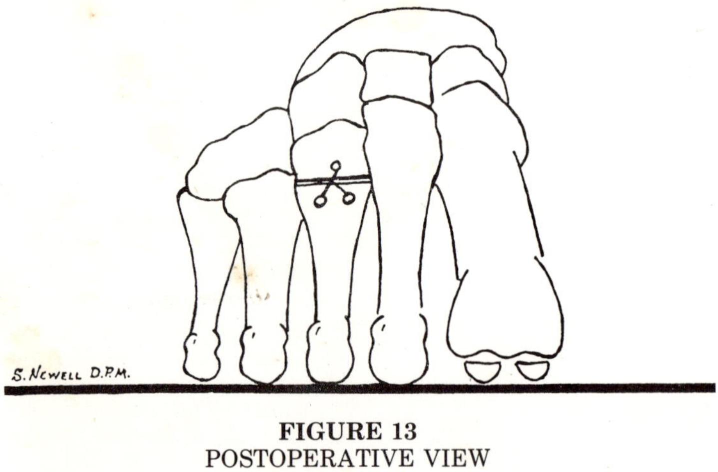

FIGURE 13
POSTOPERATIVE VIEW

The metatarsal is elevated to desired level with the foot in its functioning position and loaded.

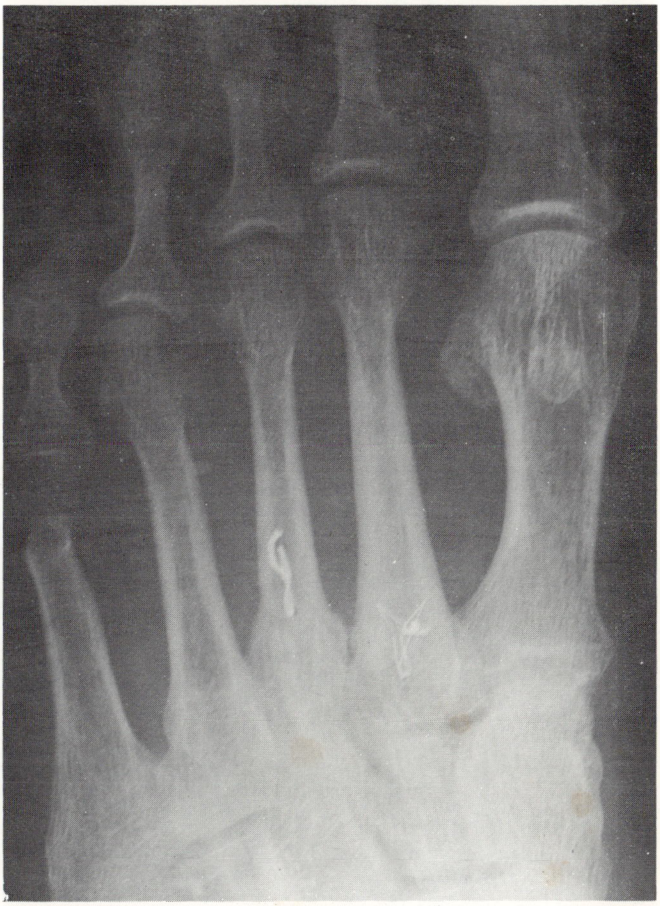

FIGURE 14
POSTOPERATIVE X-RAY

This X-ray shows good boney closure 12 weeks postoperatively.

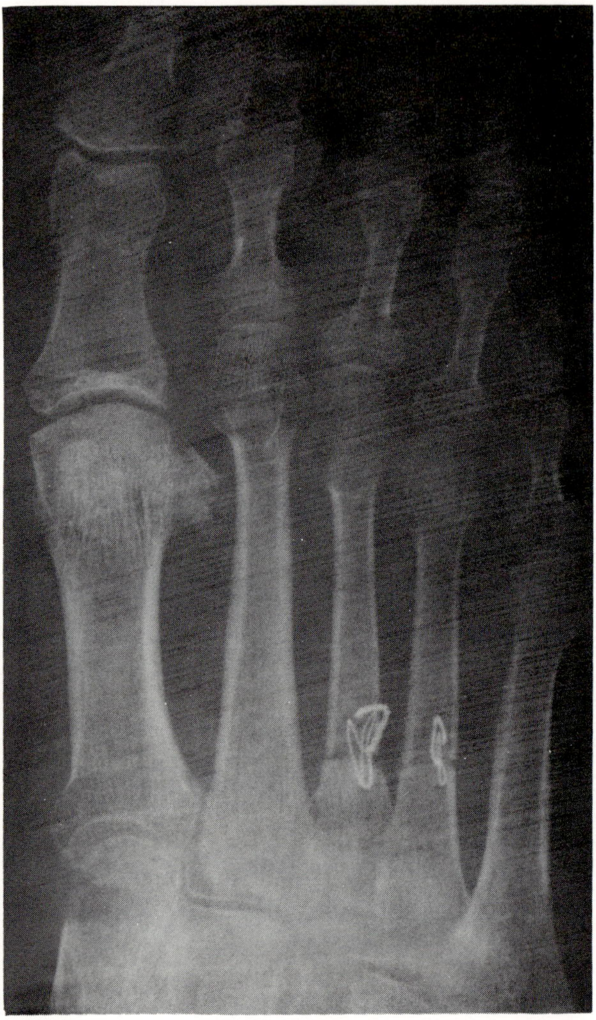

FIGURE 15
POSTOPERATIVE X-RAY

This X-ray reveals early bone absorption that sometimes presents itself in the first few weeks postoperatively on X-rays.

2. Step Down or Shortening Osteotomy

A shortening or step down osteotomy of the lesser metatarsals was first described by McKeever. However, the procedure he described was performed at the metatarsal neck. A limitation of motion at the metatarsal-phalangeal joint was a common end result. Giannestras recommended a step down osteotomy at the metatarsal base. His procedure consisted of an oblique osteotomy at the base. A hole was drilled in the proximal fragment and the distal fragment was placed in this hole. A horizontal absorbable suture was placed around the fragments. Plaster casts are not utilized following the procedure. The problem with this method is two-fold: first, the procedure is technically difficult; secondly, the amount of lengthening depends on how well the distal fragment fits into the proximal fragment. Thus, this is not the recommended method for shortening a metatarsal. The purpose of this type of procedure is to shorten a long metatarsal. As a result of the shortening, the bone is also placed on a higher plane relative to the adjacent metatarsals.

Preoperative Signs

1. A nucleated plantar keratoma is present under the 2nd, 3rd, or 4th metatarsal heads.
2. The involved metatarsal may appear prominent in relation to the adjacent metatarsals.
3. Dorsally dislocated toe may be present.
4. Long digit may be present.
5. Anterior displacement of the fat pad may be present.
6. Adequate and free range of motion at the metatarsal-phalangeal joint.

Preoperative Symptoms

1. Pain with direct or lateral pressure to the keratoma.
2. Pain, plantar aspect of metatarsal on ambulation with or without foot gear.
3. Pain when walking bare foot on a hard surface.
4. Patient may complain of a dorsally contracted toe.
5. Patient may complain of long digits.
6. Patient may complain of walking on a bone or a pebble.

Preoperative X-ray Evaluation

1. No degenerative changes of metatarsal-phalangeal joint.
2. Metatarsal should be of normal bone density.
3. The metatarsal should be longer than adjacent metatarsals.
4. Digit may appear longer than others on X-ray.
5. Dorsally located toe may be present.
6. Metatarsal may appear depressed compared to adjacent bones on axial view.

Biomechanical Evaluation

1. May be performed in presence of uncontrollable pronatory forces.
2. Postoperative orthotic control should be utilized if necessary.

Surgical Procedure

A three to four centimeter dorsal linear incision is made over the shaft of the involved metatarsal. This is deepened by sharp dissection. The extensor tendon is freed and retracted. The interossei muscles are mobilized so that the shaft of the metatarsal may be visualized. An incision is made through the periosteum which is then dissected free from the metatarsal. The osteotomy should be performed as far proximally as possible. A cut is made perpendicular to the shaft that transects the bone. A second cut is made at the predetermined site and the intervening section of bone removed. The two ends of the shaft are coaptated. If there is a problem in this maneuver, the tissue around the metatarsal shaft and the metatarsal head must be freed to allow the two ends to come together. Drill holes are placed on either side of the osteotomy site from the dorsal to the plantar surface. Twenty-eight gauge (2-0) monofilament wire is placed through the holes and tightened to keep the osteotomy in place. Intramedullary wires have been described previously in the literature to fix the osteotomy site. The two disadvantages of this type of fixation are the lack of compression of the fragments and the possible rotation of the fragments. The periosteum, subcutaneous tissue and the skin are closed in the usual manner.

Postoperative Management

The patient is placed in a short leg walking cast and allowed to ambulate when the cast is dry, in 24 to 48 hours. The patient is seen for cast checks weekly following discharge from the hospital. The cast is removed approximately 3 weeks postoperatively and the skin sutures are removed. X-rays may be taken at this point in time. The cast is reapplied for an additional two to three weeks. After this time the cast is removed and physical therapy commences. The patient is placed in a Bevin shoe and an Ace bandage for one to two weeks. X-rays are taken when the cast is removed. Orthotic control is instituted when the patient returns to regular foot gear in approximately seven to eight weeks.

Advantages

1. The primary osseous deformity is reduced.
2. The intrinsic stability of the metatarsal-phalangeal joint is maintained.
3. The metatarsal is shortened.
4. The ability to calculate preoperatively the amount of bone to be removed.

Disadvantages

1. Internal fixation is necessary.
2. Plaster immobilization is required.
3. Prolonged disability and inconvenience for the patient is required.
4. Distraction of the osteotomy site is possible which could result in poor alignment of the metatarsal, creating new symptomatology.
5. Osteoporosis may ensue.
6. Care must be taken to properly use the power equipment.
7. Complete transection of the bone creates a very unstable situation.
8. If too much bone is removed, the fragments may not be able to be brought together.

A. The normal metatarsal parabola is drawn connecting the metatarsal heads. As is noted in this illustration the third metatarsal is longer than any of the others. The amount of this length discrepancy may be measured and used to determine the amount of bone to be resected.

B. A dorsal view showing the section of bone resected from the proximal portion of the metatarsal. The placement of the two drill holes for the wire fixation is shown.

C. The through-and-through dorsal-planter wire fixation is demonstrated. The two portions of bone are brought together to shorten the metatarsal.

D. In this case the cut of the distal piece is angled to allow dorsiflexion as well as shortening of the metatarsal. It should be noted that shortening the metatarsal also allows for a slight amount of dorsiflexion.

E. Following the shortening of the metatarsal the entire metatarsal parabol returns to a normal configuration.

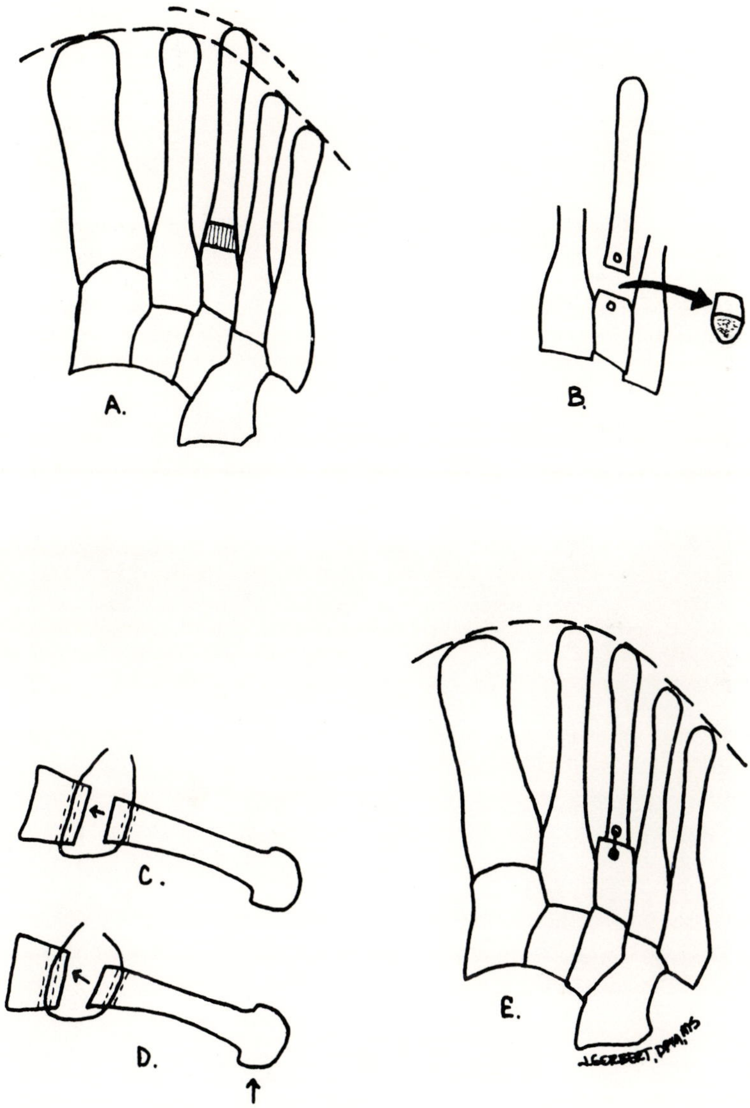

FIGURE 1
SHORTENING PROCEDURE

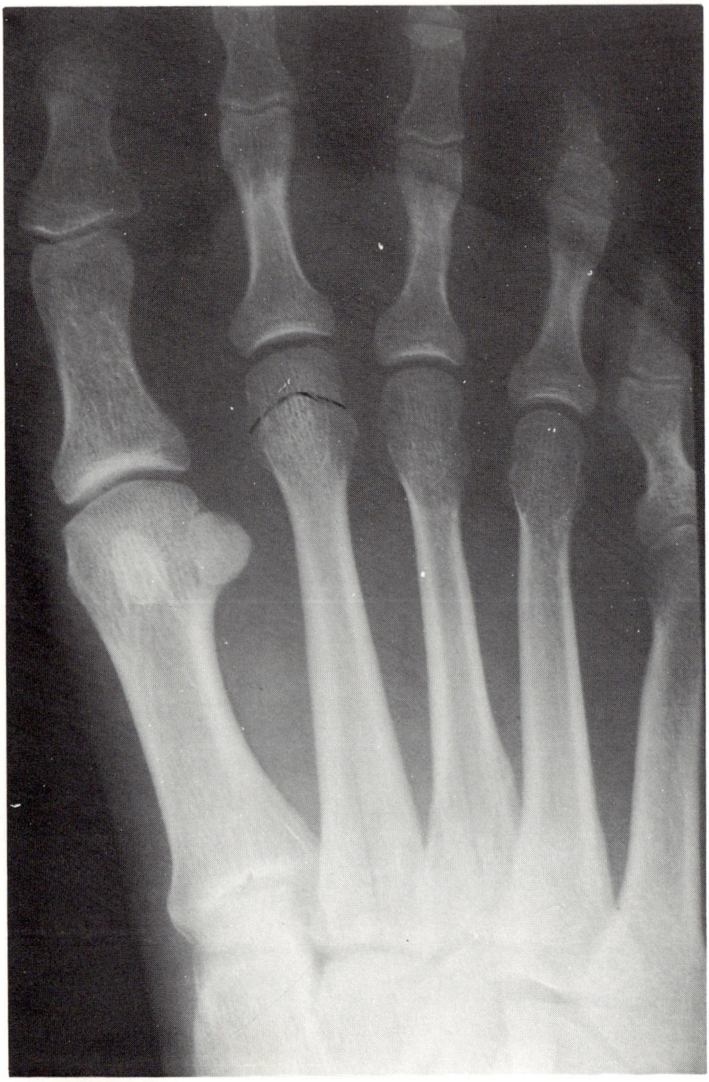

FIGURE 2A
PREOPERATIVE AP X-RAY

Preoperative AP showing abnormal metatarsal pattern. The dotted line represents the position of the metatarsal head following the procedure.

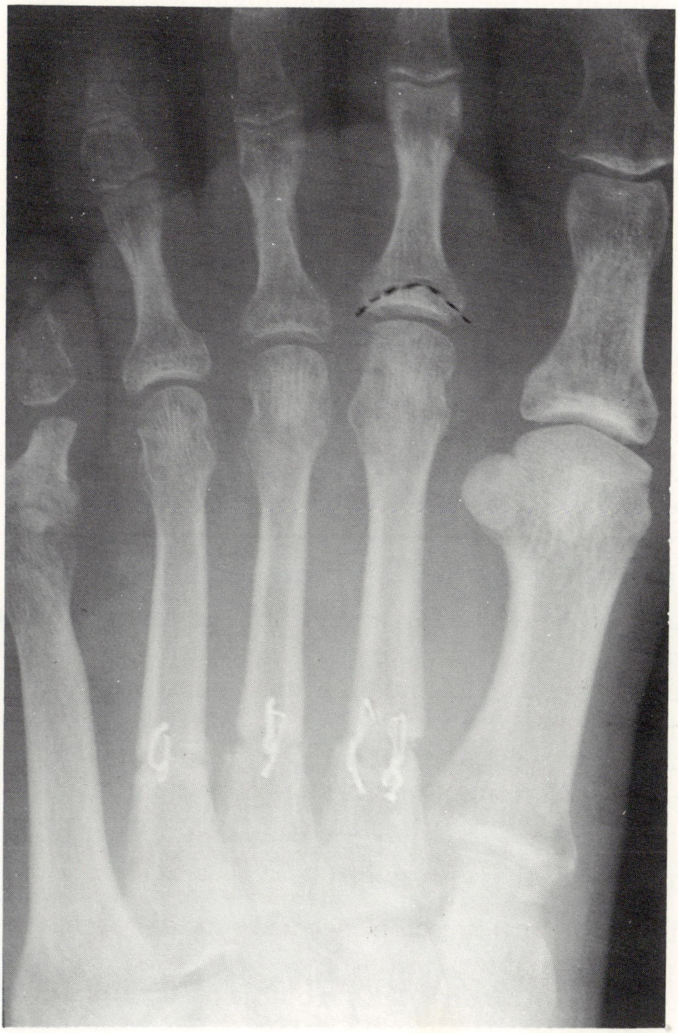

FIGURE 2B
POSTOPERATIVE AP X-RAY

Postoperative AP showing the osteotomy site fixed with 2-0 monofilament steel suture. The dotted line in this X-ray represents the position of the head preoperatively.

3. Extension Osteoarthrotomy (E.O.A.)

This procedure involves the resection of the base of a lesser metatarsal (2, 3, or 4) in a wedge shape manner so as to allow dorsiflexion of the metatarsal upon weight bearing. It is used for correction of a depressed metatarsal associated with an intractable plantar keratoma, especially in the aged patient where immobilization and internal or external fixation are not desired.

Preoperative Signs

1. An intractable plantar keratoma is present under the involved metatarsal head.
2. The metatarsal head is prominent when the foot is placed in a loaded position and palpated plantarly as compared to the other metatarsal heads.
3. The range of motion of the involved metatarsal-phalangeal joint should be adequate and without crepitation.
4. The involved ray may have an associated dorsally contracted toe.

Preoperative Symptoms

1. Pain in the involved area with ambulation in most foot gear.
2. Pain upon direct pressure to the plantar lesion.
3. The patient may complain of discomfort when ambulating without shoes.
4. No pain when the involved metatarsal-phalangeal joint is taken through its normal range of motion.

Biomechanical Evaluation

1. This procedure can be performed in the presence of uncontrollable pronatory forces.
2. Some form of an orthotic is required postoperatively which is usually of the accomodative type.

Preoperative X-ray Evaluation

1. The metatarsal-phalangeal joint of the involved ray shows no degenerative signs.
2. The involved metatarsal head is within normal limits.
3. The involved metatarsal head appears plantarly depressed as seen on an axial view of the foot.
4. Osteoporosis may be present.
5. The metatarsal may be abnormally long.

Surgical Procedure

For this procedure the third metatarsal is used as an example. A 2.5 to 3.0 centimeter dorsilinear incision is made over the third metatarsal base — cuneiform joint. By sharp and blunt dissection the extensor digitorum longus tendon to the fourth toe and the extensor digitorum brevis tendon to the third toe are identified. The longus tendon is retracted medially and the brevis tendon is retracted laterally. Depending on how far medial the skin incision was made over the metatarsal-cuneiform joint the extensor brevis tendon to the second toe may also be visible and will be retracted, along with the longus tendon, medially. The metatarsal-cuneiform joint is palpated and a dorsal linear incision is made through the overlying soft tissue and periosteum down to bone extending over the metatarsal base, the joint, and the distal aspect of the third cuneiform. Using a sharp periosteal elevator the soft tissue is freed from the metatarsal base thereby exposing the joint. In dissection one must use extreme care to preserve the arcuate artery which crosses transversely in this area giving rise to the intermetatarsal arteries. This can be accomplished by keeping the dissection to a minimum and by using blunt instrumentation as much as possible. Using an oscillating blade on a power hand piece the base of the metatarsal is resected in a wedge shape, with the base dorsal and the apex plantar. After removing this piece of bone the ligaments around the metatarsal base which connect it to the adjacent metatarsals and to the cuneiform must be incised. If this is not performed the desired amount of dorsiflexion of the metatarsal can not be achieved. With the foot in a loaded position pressure is applied to the plantar aspect of the metatarsal head in a dorsal direction to determine if the metatarsal will move easily to the desired corrected position. If it does not then sufficient bone has not been removed and/or all of the ligaments have not been incised. It is the latter which is usually at fault. The amount of bone which usually has to be excised is 2 to 3 millimeters dorsally. When you are satisfied with the movement of the metatarsal the area is flushed with sterile saline and the soft tissue layer is closed over the metatarsal-cuneiform joint using 4-0 or 5-0 absorbable suture. The subcutaneous tissue is closed using 5-0 nylon suture. If the plantar lesion is well demarcated and fibrotic you may decide to ellipse it at this time. The postoperative dressing is of the usual gauze type. However, if the lesion was ellipsed, then a small buttress pad is place under the involved metatarsal head to elevate it to the desired position and to maintain it there, since the patient will probably remain non-weight bearing for several weeks. If the patient is allowed to ambulate then the body weight will push the metatarsal dorsal to the level of the adjacent metatarsals.

Postoperative Management

The patient is encouraged to begin ambulation as soon as possible, usually using a wooden surgical shoe. If the plantar lesion was excised then the patient is kept non-weight bearing on that foot for approximately two weeks to allow for good plantar healing without undue tension on the wound. The average hospital stay is approximately 3 days. X-rays are taken at the first dressing change, approximately seven days postoperatively. The dorsal sutures are removed at the second dressing change, approximately fourteen days postoperatively. The plantar sutures, if the lesion was ellipsed, are removed at the third dressing change, approximately twenty-one days postoperatively. Orthotics are constructed at this time and the patient can usually return to regular shoes in 3 to 4 weeks postoperatively. The dorsal edema which usually develops to some extent can be controlled with physical therapy, elevation of the involved foot and leg, and restriction of prolonged standing or dependent position of the foot.

Advantages

1. Preserves the metatarsal-phalangeal joint.
2. Does not require internal or external fixation.
3. Shorter disability postoperatively than most osteotomy procedures which require immobilization.
4. Requires no immobilization.
5. Does not require a time period for osseous healing.
6. Can be performed in the geriatric patient.

Disadvantages

1. No accurate method for determining the amount of bone to be resected.
2. Dorsiflexion of the metatarsal relies on external pressure postoperatively.
3. Arthritic changes may occur where the metatarsal base was resected with resultant postoperative discomfort in this area with ambulation.

4. Improper surgical technique may result in an inadequate positioned metatarsal head.
5. A painful pseudoarthrosis may result at the metatarsal-cuneiform articulation.

A. This diagram shows an axial type view of the forefoot demonstrating a depressed third metatarsal. The shaded area at the base of the metatarsal represents the amount of bone which is to be resected.

B. This is a sagittal view of the third metatarsal and third cuneiform showing the shape and amount of bone which is to be resected from the base of the metatarsal. Note the triangular shape to the bone that is to be resected with its base dorsal and its apex plantar.

C. This is a sagittal view after the bone has been resected showing how the metatarsal is dorsiflexed and also slightly shortened.

D. This diagram is an axial type view of the forefoot after the base of the metatarsal has been resected and before any pressure is applied to the metatarsal head to dorsiflex it.

E. This is a dorsal view of the metatarsal and cuneiform demonstrating how the ligaments which connect the metatarsal to the adjacent metatarsals and to the cuneiform must be incised in order to achieve freedom of motion of the metatarsal. When actually performing this step of the surgical procedure one should keep the blade next to the metatarsal bone at all times in order to keep the trauma to a minimum.

F. This is an axial type view following the procedure showing how external pressure to the plantar aspect of the foot will elevate the metatarsal to its desired position.

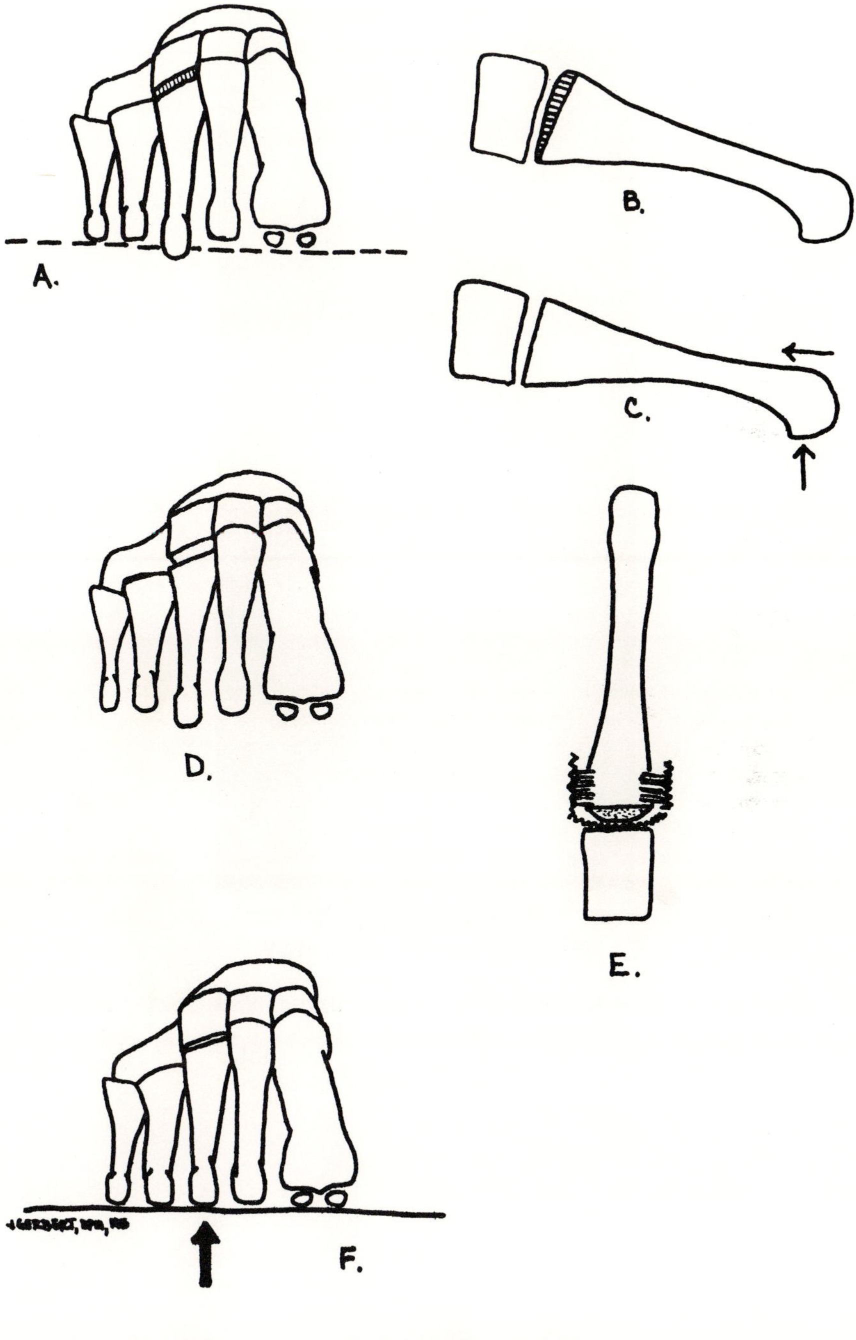

FIGURE 1
EXTENSION OSTEOARTHROTOMY (EOA)

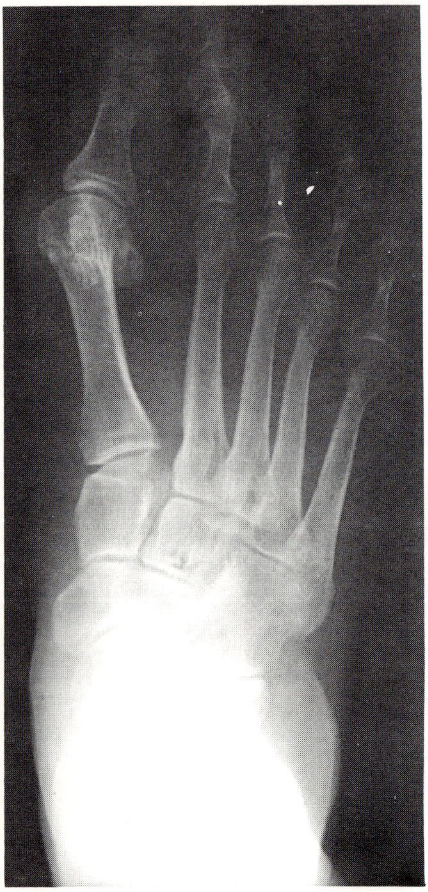

FIGURE 2A
PREOPERATIVE A-P X-RAY

Note the normal appearing 2nd metatarsal-2nd cuneiform joint. Clinically, the patient had an intractable plantar keratoma sub-2nd metatarsal head.

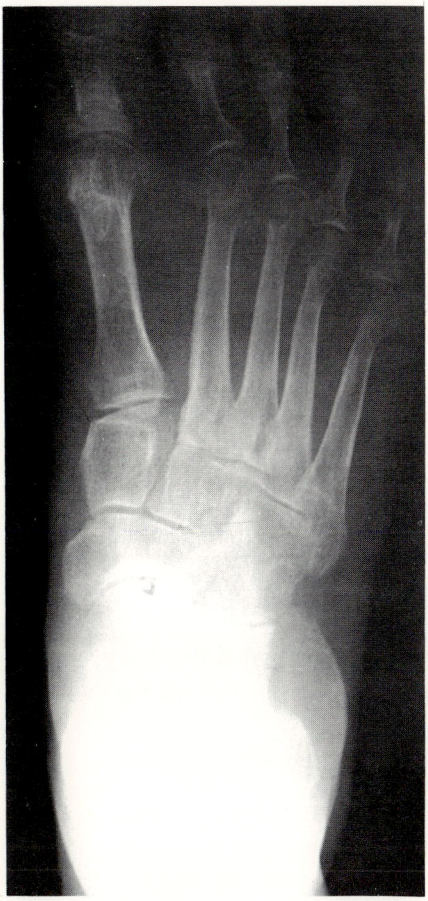

FIGURE 2B
POSTOPERATIVE A-P X-RAY

This is a postoperative X-ray following an extension osteoarthrotomy of the second metatarsal. No fixation is required. Note the closed 2nd metatarsal-2nd cuneiform joint due to dorsiflexion of the metatarsal.

4. Crescentic Osteotomy

Use of lesser metatarsal crescentic osteotomies for Intractable Plantar Keratoses (IPK) correction alone is rare. The main use of the crescentic osteotomy is to correct a transverse plane deviation of abductus or adductus. However, when the patient presents a combined deformity usually involving both transverse and sagittal plane abormalities, then a lesser metatarsal crescentic osteotomy is indicated.

Preoperative Signs

1. Fibrous shearing callous (non-nucleated).
2. Dorsally dislocated digit, but not subluxed.
3. Plantarly prominent metatarsal.

Preoperative Symptoms

1. Pain in shoes and weight bearing.
2. No pain out of shoes.
3. Burning sensation in callous.

Biomechanical Evaluation

1. Minimal biomechanical deformity, usually forefoot varus.
2. Equinus is an inconstant finding.

Pre-Operative X-ray Evaluation

1. Minimal length increase in metatarsal.
2. No joint disease present.

Surgical Procedure

The skin incision is placed directly over the base area of the metatarsal if a single osteotomy is performed, or between adjacent metatarsals if multiple osteotomies are to be performed. The skin incision is carried from mid-shaft of the metatarsal to beyond the metatarso-cuneiform joint.

The subcutaneous tissue is dissected free to expose the extensor tendons and their sheaths. Blunt dissection may be employed in an effort to identify the medial aspect and lateral margin of the metatarsal. Once these margins are identified, sharp dissection is utilized to mobilize the extensor tendons from the base area of the metatarsal.

Once the dorsal surface of the metatarsal is exposed, the dorsal interossei muscles must be sharply dissected from the sides of the metatarsals where they originate. This will enable placement of retractors that serve both to expose the metatarsal on three sides, and to protect the adjacent soft tissue from the power equipment.

The osteotomy is then performed employing either a power drill or a crescentic blade on an oscillating saw. The cut is made from the dorsum to the plantar and is complete. The cut is concave with the dome facing proximally.

Closure of the subcutaneous and skin structures is delayed until all the metatarsal osteotomies are performed.

Fixation of lesser metatarsal crescentic osteotomies is usually not necessary since this procedure is usually employed in conjunction with pan metatarsal osteotomies.

Position of the lesser metatarsal crescentic osteotomy is maintained by plaster casts. Separate wire fixation is not necessary.

Postoperative Management

Postoperative shoes are most often used for postoperative control, occasionally an ambulatory slipper cast may be used for a 4-6 week period. Shoe wearing may begin soon after edema is controlled.

Advantages

1. Useful in combined deformities adductus and plantar flexion.
2. Excellent procedure where length must be maintained.

Disadvantages

1. Not useful in severe nucleated intractable plantar keratomas.

This represents crescentic osteotomy of the lesser metatarsals. The cut is made approximately one centimeter from the metatarsal cuneiform joint.

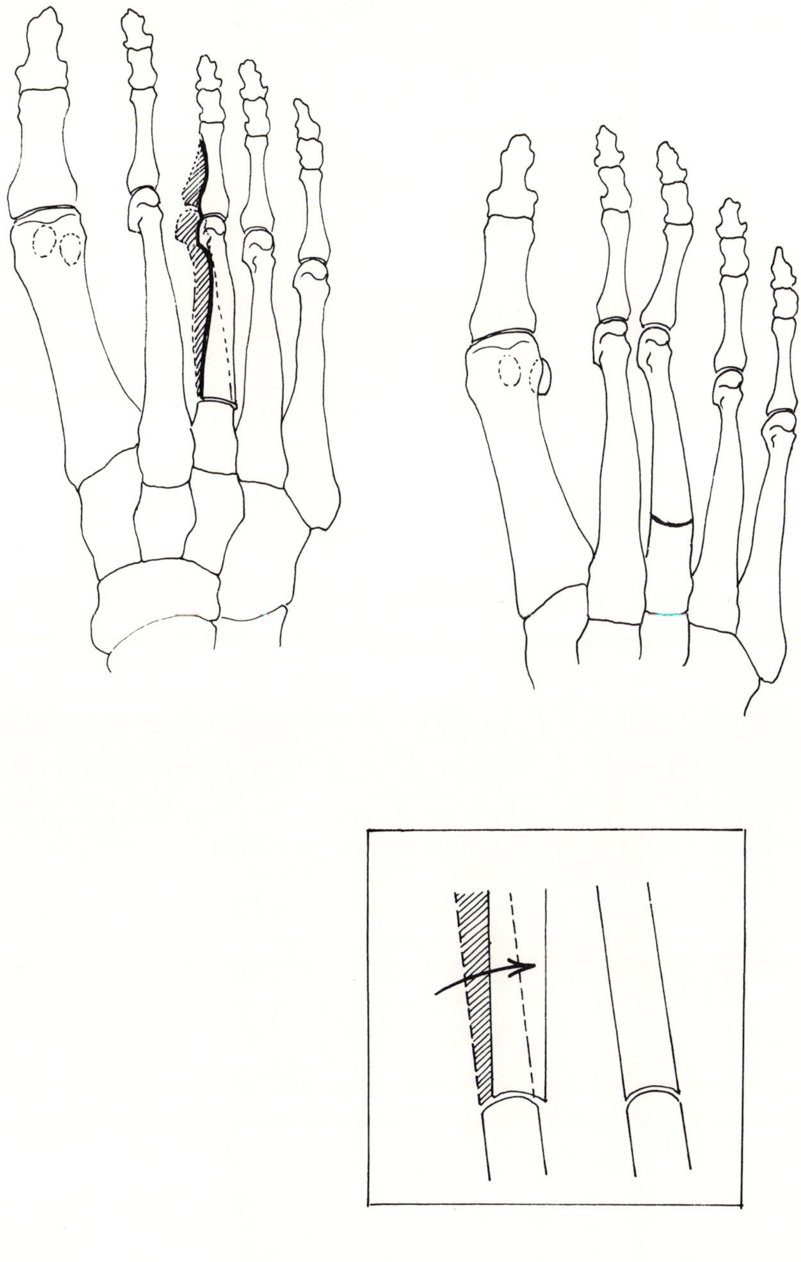

FIGURE 1
CRESCENTIC OSTEOTOMY

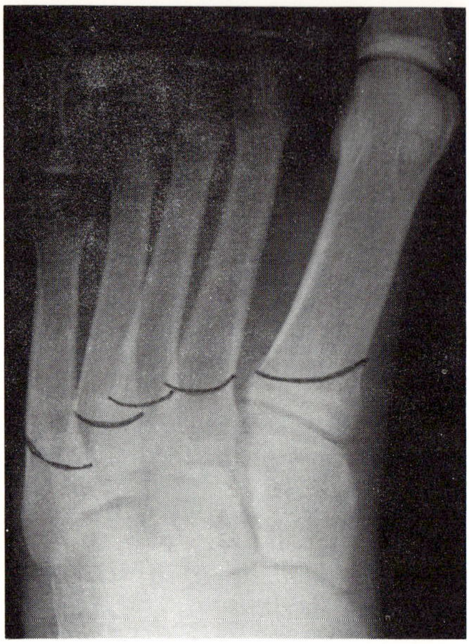

FIGURE 2A
PREOPERATIVE X-RAY

Preoperative determination for crescentic osteotomies to be performed on the bases of the metatarsals.

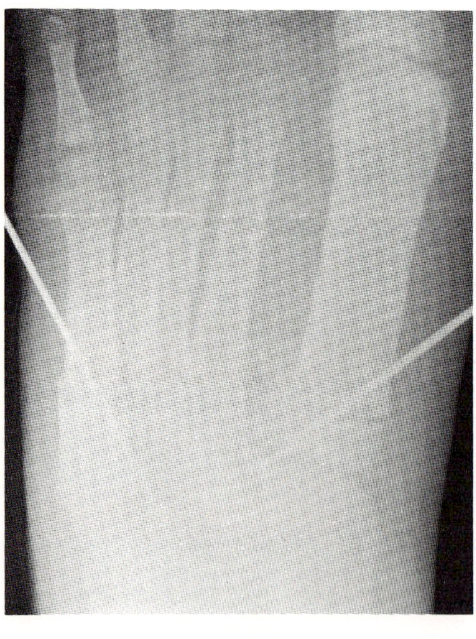

FIGURE 2B
POSTOPERATIVE X-RAY

K-wiring of the metatarsals.

5. Osteoclasis-type Procedures

a. V-Osteotomy at Neck of Metatarsal

This procedure was first described by Jacoby in 1973. The procedure is a variant of other osteotomies that have been performed at the metatarsal neck. The purpose of the procedure is to raise the level of the metatarsal head while preventing medial or lateral shift of the distal fragment. Fixation is not used as the metatarsal head is left free to seek its own level.

Preoperative Signs

1. A nucleated plantar keratoma is present under the 2nd, 3rd, or 4th metatarsal.
2. The involved metatarsal may appear prominent in relation to the adjacent metatarsals.
3. Adequate and free range of motion should exist at the metatarso-phalangeal joint.
4. Dorsally located toe may be present.
5. Long digit may be present.

Preoperative Symptoms

1. Pain with direct or lateral pressure to the keratoma.
2. Pain plantar aspect of metatarsal on ambulation with or without foot gear.
3. Pain especially when walking bare foot on a hard surface.
4. Patient may complain of dorsally contracted toe.
5. Patient may complain of long digit.

Preoperative X-ray Evaluation

1. No degenerative changes of the metatarsal phalangeal joint.
2. Metatarsal may appear depressed in relation to other metatarsals on an axial view.
3. Metatarsal may appear longer than adjacent metatarsals.
4. Digit may appear longer than others on X-ray.
5. Dorsally located toe may be present.
6. Metatarsal should be of normal bone density.

Biomechanical Evaluation

1. May be performed in the presence of uncontrollable pronatory forces.
2. Postoperative orthotic control should be utilized if necessary.

Surgical Procedure

A three to four centimeter dorsal linear incision is made over the distal portion of the metatarsal. As the incision is deepened the extensor longus and brevis tendons are identified and retracted laterally. The tissue surrounding the metatarsal neck is reflected for exposure of the bone. With a power oscillating saw a "V" osteotomy is made at the surgical neck. The apex of the "V" is directed distally. The osteotomy may be made with or without leaving the plantar cortex intact. The advantage of not cutting the plantar cortex is to keep the metatarsal head from moving too high. The advantages of a complete osteotomy are two fold: first there is less pain noticed postoperatively by the patient; second, one is more certain that the metatarsal head will seek its proper level and will not be held by any bony attachments. Once the osteotomy is made the distal fragments is manually pushed upward to impact with the metatarsal shaft. The deep tissues are closed with absorbable suture followed by normal skin closure.

Postoperative Management

A sterile compression dressing is applied following surgery. The patient is placed in a wooden postoperative shoe and ambulation is allowed immediately. The sutures are removed 10 days to 2 weeks post-operatively. At this time postoperative X-rays are taken and the patient is allowed to return to normal shoe gear.

Advantages

1. The intrinsic stability of the metatarso-phalangeal joint is maintained.
2. The procedure does not require the removal of any bone.
3. Minimal disability results from this procedure.
4. Postoperative casts are not necessary.
5. An attempt is made to stop lateral dislocation of the metatarsal head.

Disadvantages

1. Non-union may occur.
2. Swelling may remain for a longer period of time than usual.
3. If the metatarsal moves too high a transfer lesion may occur.
4. Care must be taken to properly perform the osteotomy with the power equipment.
5. The metatarsal head may not move dorsal enough because of the intact plantar cortex.

6. A decrease of motion at the metatarsal-phalangeal joint is possible.
7. A dorsal prominence may occur as a result of the callus.

This figure demonstrates the various steps in performing a "V" osteotomy at the metatarsal neck.

A. This is a dorsal view showing the manner in which the metatarsal will be sectioned.

B. Another dorsal view after the osteotomy is completed.

C. This is a lateral view demonstrating the cut in the bone. The dotted line represents the apex of the "V".

D. This lateral view shows the impaction of the head into the shaft as the metatarsal is raised. One can also note the amount of dorsiflexion that one can obtain.

E. The final position of the metatarsal is noted. One can note a slight dorsal prominence may be present.

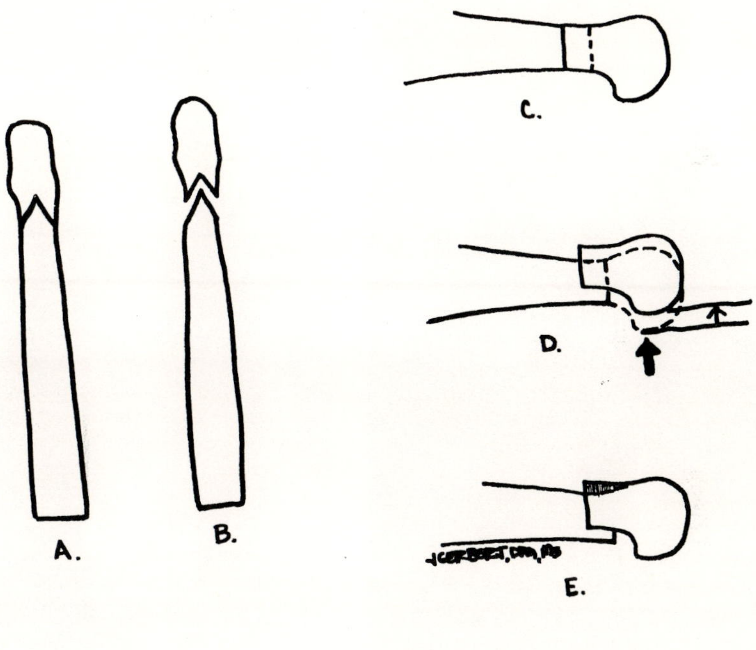

FIGURE 1
V-OSTEOTOMY AT NECK OF METATARSAL

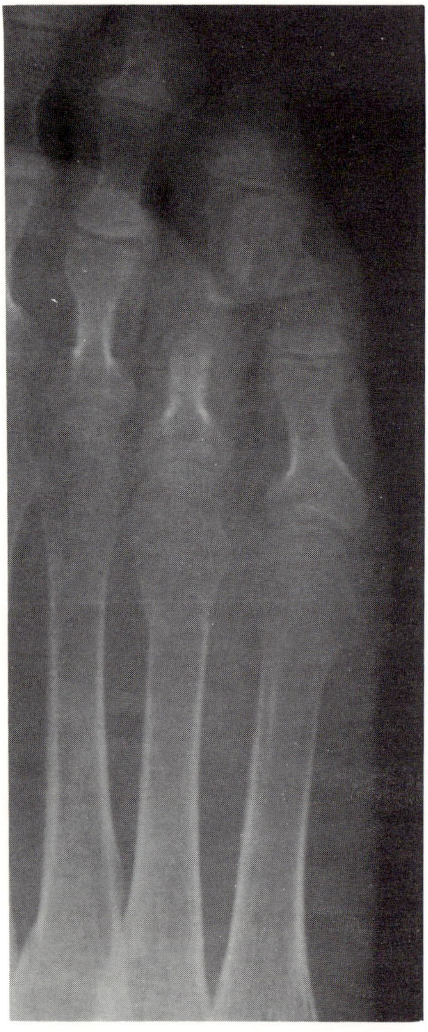

FIGURE 2A
PREOPERATIVE A-P X-RAY

This is a preoperative A-P view. The 4th metatarsal phalangeal is normal in appearance. The range of motion is adequate with no pain. The osteotomy will be performed in the metahyseal area of the neck, just proximal to the capsule.

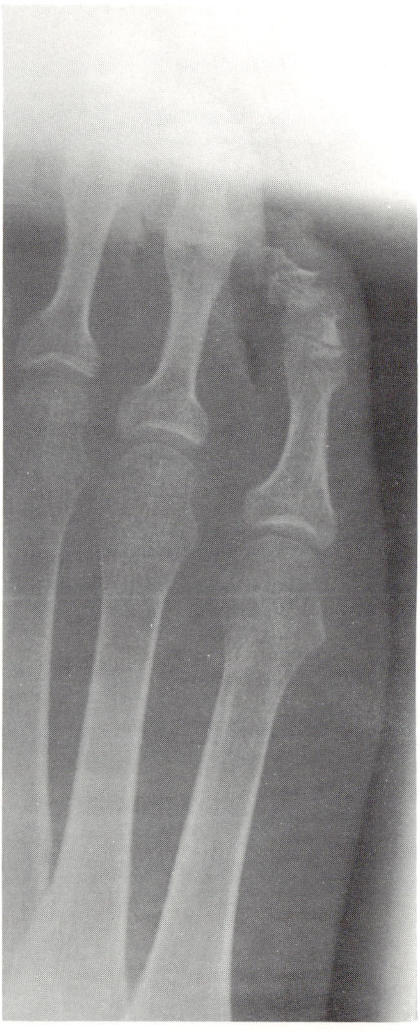

FIGURE 2 B
POSTOPERATIVE A-P X-RAY

Note the position of the osteotomy in the neck of the metatarsal. The cut is in the shape of the "V" with the apex facing distally. The head is then impacted into the shaft of the metatarsal.

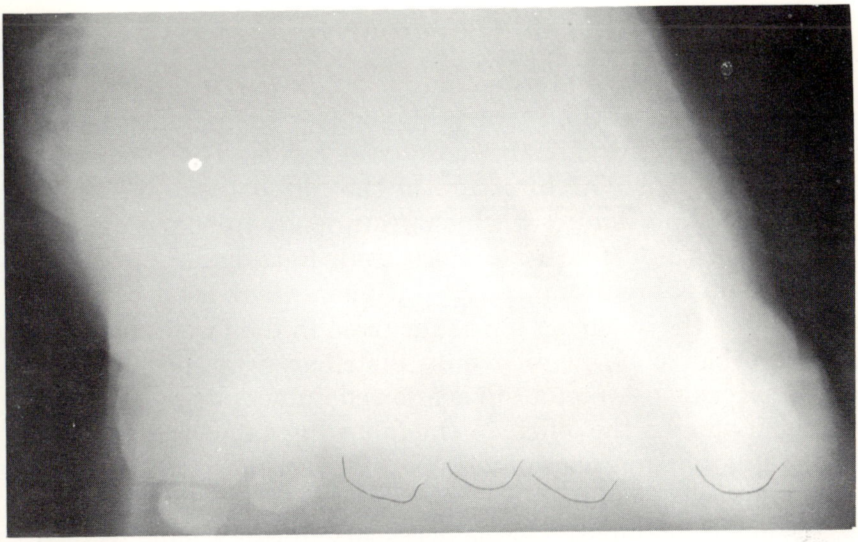

FIGURE 3A
PREOPERATIVE AXIAL X-RAY

The preoperative axial X-ray shows a depression of the fourth metatarsal. The plantar condyles are normal and do not appear prominent.

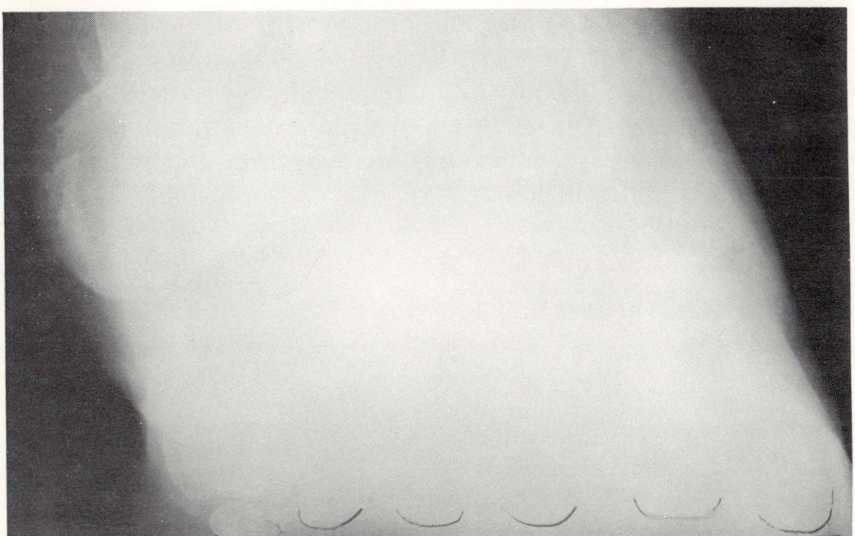

FIGURE 3B
POSTOPERATIVE AXIAL X-RAY

The postoperative axial view shows the amount that the fourth metatarsal has been raised. In this case we can see that it is above the level of the third metatarsal.

b. Open Metaphyseal Osteotomy

The open metaphyseal osteotomy is a new surgical technique for the treatment of the intractable plantar keratoma beneath the second, third, or fourth metatarsal heads. The technique maintains the basic architecture of the forefoot and offers an uncomplicated procedure in which a surgically freed metatarsal head will seek and find its proper level. Retrograde forces incurred during ambulation force the metatarsal head dorsally which allows the shearing forces incurred in the forefoot during the gait cycle to be more evenly distributed to the adjacent metatarsal heads. Ambulation is allowed immediately following surgery, if done in the office, or the following day if peformed in the hospital. Long periods of postoperative care are unnecessary as are long periods of medication following surgery. A minimal amount of surgical dissection is necessary in this simple technique to attain good results commonly in the 80 percentile range.

The surgical technique described in this chapter uses the Lombodi osteotome and the Rush mallet. Other instruments are commonly used by many podiatric surgeons to accomplish the same end result of allowing the freed metatarsal head to seek its own level. These instruments can be either manual or power equipment. The various manual bone cutting instruments can be used, as well as power equipment such as the Stryker reciprocating bone saw, the Ritter, Hall, White, Emsco, Foredom, or Dremel power drills using the Lindner, Prober, or Shannon burrs. It is most important to note that the angle of cut goes dorsally from distal to proximal, as illustrated in Figure 1. This is done to prevent the metatarsal head from going to high, causing a dorsal 'bump' and a transfer lesion.

Preoperative Signs

1. Plantar keratoma (nucleated or non-nucleated) beneath a lessor metatarsal head.
2. Depressed metatarsal head in relation to other metatarsal heads.
3. Axial view X-rays indicate a sublocated metatarsal head.
4. Dorsally subluxed proximal phalanx of the affected ray.
5. Localized inflammation in any stage beneath the affected ray.
6. Pathomechanical foot.
7. Enlarged metatarsal head or condyles (not Freibergs).
8. Capsulitis of affected metatarsal phalangeal joint.

Preoperative Symptoms

1. Sharp pain on ambulation beneath the affected metatarsal head.
2. Sharp pain upon direct palpation of the lesion.
3. Compensation of affected foot during stance phase of gait.
4. Pain in legs, thigh, or low back from accommodative gait.
5. Tenderness around affected metatarsal-phalangeal joint.

Preoperative X-ray Evaluation

1. No visualization of keratoma on X-ray. (Wire lesions to locate.)
2. Metatarsal head may be enlarged.
3. Excessive metatarsal length.
4. Axial views usually show sublocated metatarsal head in relation to adjacent metatarsal heads.
5. Subluxed metatarsal phalangeal joint may be visualized.
6. Normal metatarsal phalangeal articulation visualized on dorsal-plantar view.
7. Closure of the epiphysis of the lesser metatarsals should be present.

Biomechanical Evaluation

The contact period in a compensated forefoot varus is generally lengthened by pronation of the subtalar articulation and the midtarsal articulations. Pronation extends this period until the forefoot is able to compensate to reach the supportive surface. Therefore the foot is pronated and mobile at a time when it should be becoming supinated and rigid. In the young with good muscle power the pronation may be overcome, but with fatigue and age the foot is only able to reach a supinated attitude during the swing phase. With pronation of the subtalar articulations and the midtarsal articulations, the 1st ray becomes hypermobile, a shearing force is developed under the second metatarsal head with development of a nucleated plantar keratoma.

Any pathomechanical foot in which there is untimely pronation of the subtalar articulations or midtarsal articulations, 1st or 5th rays, creates excess motion of the metatarsals when they should be fixed rigid lever arms for proper propulsion. The metatarsals have abnormal movement, while the skin is fixed by friction to the weightbearing surface, creating a shearing force in the transverse plane. The shearing force is compounded proportionately to the increase in mobility of the forefoot. Foot types on which plantar keratomas appear include forefoot varus, forefoot valgus, triceps surae equinus, and rearfoot varus.

Surgical Procedure

The open metaphyseal osteotomy should not be performed unless the proximal phalanx can be manipulated distally off the metatarsal head and maintained in this position with the foot loaded.

A linear longitudinal incision approximately 3 cm in length is made over the affected metatarsal medial to the extensor tendons. The incision commences at the metatarsal phalangeal articulation and extends proximally. The incision is deepened through subcutaneous tissue, and the tendons of extensor digitorum longus and extensor digitorum brevis are exposed. The tendons are then retracted medially or laterally with a small Weitlander retractor. Thus is exposed the dorsal aspect of the neck of the metatarsal and most dorsal proximal aspect of the metatarsal head. With minimal dissection, the sides of the distal aspect of the metatarsal neck is exposed scoring the bone to be cut. A 2″ x 4″ x 1″ autoclaved wooden block is then held beneath the plantar forefoot to support the metatarsal parabola solidly during the osteotomy. With a 16 oz. Rush mallet and a 1 cm. Lombodi osteotome held perpendicular to the long axis of the metatarsal, the shaft is transsected at the metaphysis (anatomical neck) freeing the metatarsal head from the shaft. The head is not fixed, but allowed to seek its proper level upon ambulation. The plantar aspect of the intact metatarsal shaft is then inspected carefully to be certain there are no protruding osseous plantar features still present other then normal metatarsal shaft. The retractor is then released and the vital structures realigned. The extensor tendons are then identified and may be lengthened using "Z" tendon slides if desired. The surgical site may then be closed with 2-0 Dexon sutures subcutaneously if subcutaneous sutures seem to be necessary. The skin is opposed and maintained with interrupted 5-0 nylon sutures. ½ cc of Decadron is then injected into the osteotomy site following closure. Adaptic is then placed over the surgical site and maintained in place with sterile compression dressings of four 4 x 4 gauze sponges over the dorsal incision site held in place with 1 roll of sterile 2″ Kling, with no plantar padding, around the forefoot.

Postoperative Management

1. Sterile compression dressing.
2. 24 hour ambulation to allow head to seek its proper level dorsally.

3. Reece shoe for 2-3 weeks following surgery to affected foot.
4. Analgesic of choice.
5. Postoperative X-rays at 10 days to assure alignment.
6. Weekly visits to office following surgery for 5 weeks, then once a month for 2 months.
7. Suture removal at 14-21 days.
8. Follow with biomechanical exam and fabrication of orthotics.

Advantages

1. Visualization of bone to be surgerized.
2. Maintenance of length pattern of metatarsal parabola.
3. Maintenance of proper spacing between metatarsal heads, as opposed to a metatarsal head resection.
4. Technique is simpler than most other metatarsal osteotomies.
5. No casting necessary.
6. Patient may ambulate immediately after surgery in surgical shoe.
7. Painful intractible plantar keratomas will disappear within 3 to 12 weeks following surgery.
8. Technique is easily performed in office.
9. Minimal swelling and bone callous with steroid injected into osteotomy site. Some patients require no analgesic following steroid injection into surgical site.

Disadvantages

1. Abnormal displacement of head may occur with short immobilization.
2. Pseudoarthrosis.
3. Rotation of head may cause pain.
4. Infection.
5. Excessive dorsal swelling.
6. Allergic reaction to suture material.
7. Non-union or delayed union from improper or abbreviated immobilization in surgical shoes.
8. Not to be performed on subluxed metatarsal-phalangeal joints. Where the subluxation will restrict the dorsal movement of the metatarsal other techniques should be considered.
9. No change in position of metatarsal head.
   COMMENT: It cannot be over emphasized that the patient must walk on the surgerized foot (feet) to allow the retrograde forces of the weight bearing surface to move the freed metatarsal head dorsally.
10. Transfer lesions.

A-C illustrate an open metaphyseal osteotomy of either the 2nd, 3rd or 4th metatarsals, using the Lombodi osteotme and mallet. D shows that after the metaphyseal osteotomy, upon weight bearing, the metatarsal seeks its own level in alignment with adjacent metatarsals.

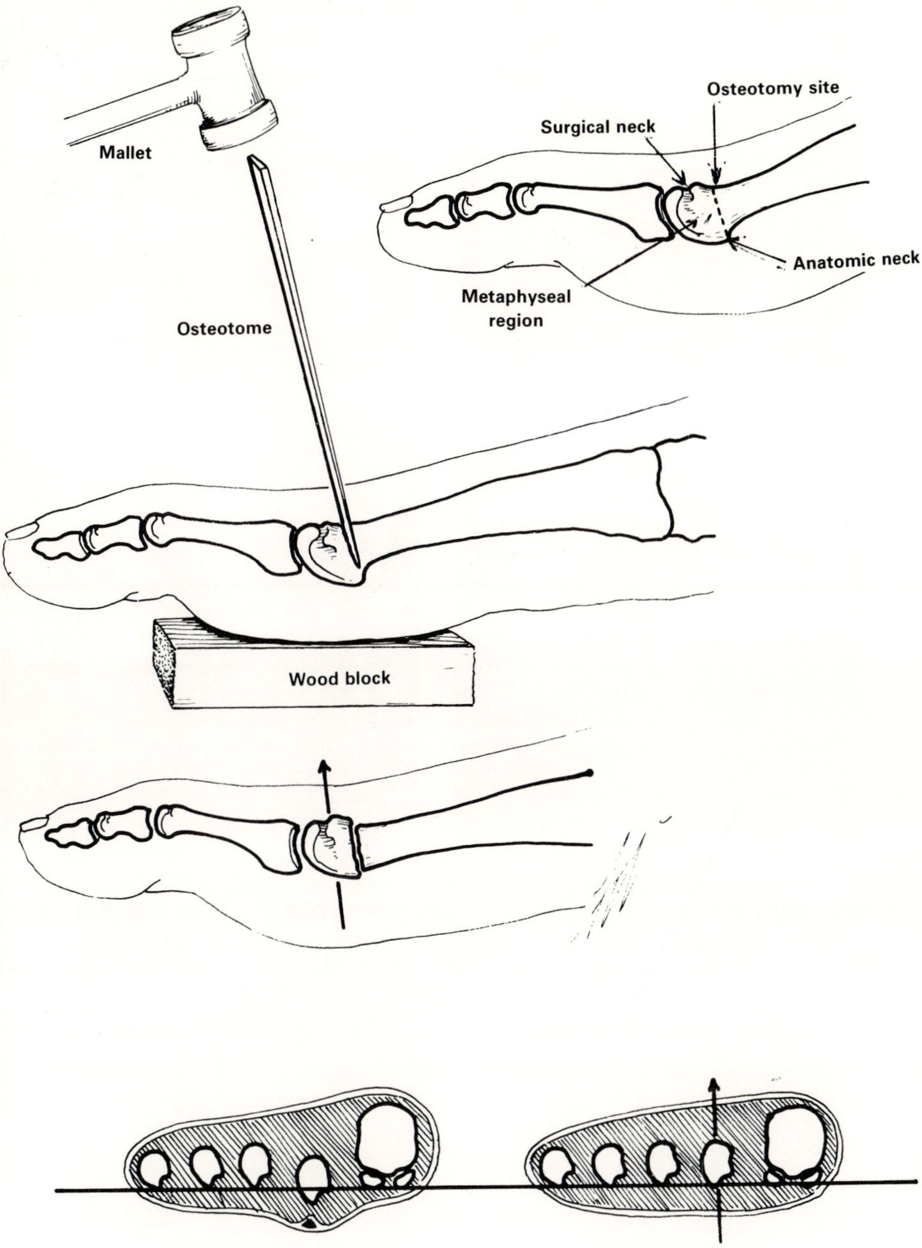

FIGURE 1
OPEN METAPHSEAL OSTEOTOMY

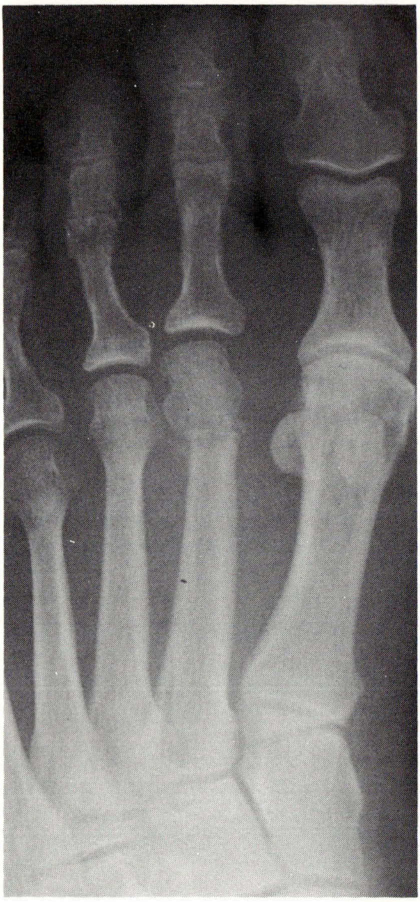

FIGURE 2A
PREOPERATIVE A-P X-RAY

Open Metaphyseal Osteotomy 2nd Metatarsal Head.

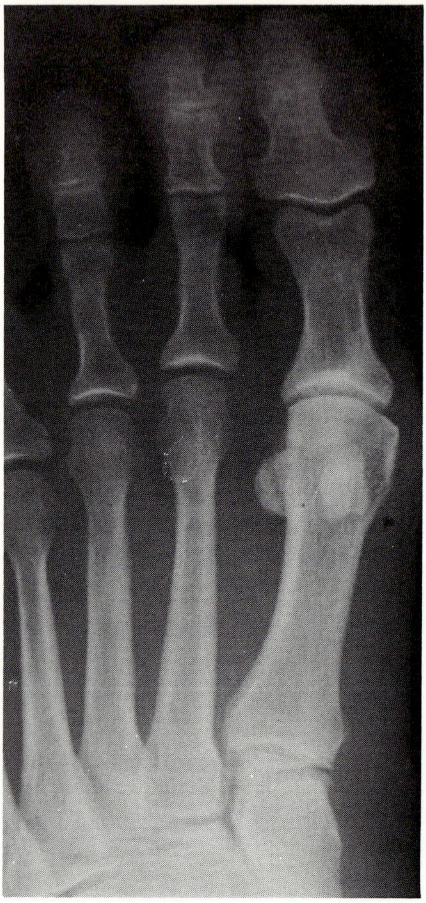

FIGURE 2B
POSTOPERATIVE A-P X-RAY

Open Metaphyseal Osteotomy 2nd Metatarsal Head.

6. Plantar Condylectomy

The plantar condylectomy was first described by Dr. Henry DuVries to eradicate plantar keratomas. The original procedure removed only the plantar condyles of the metatarsal head. Eventually the procedure also included resection the anterior one-third of the metatarsal head. Dr. DuVries claimed better results with this later method of performing the operation. The purpose of the procedure is to remove a prominent condyle that is causing a plantar keratoma. The fibular condyle is usually the source of the problem due to the rotation at the metatarsal head.

Preoperative Signs

1. A nucleated plantar keratoma is present under the 2nd, 3rd, or 4th metatarsal head.
2. The metatarsal head can be palpated and appears prominent in relation to the adjacent metatarsal heads.
3. Dorsally located toe may be present.
4. Hammer toe may be present.
5. Anterior displacement of the fat pad may be present.

Preoperative Symptoms

1. Pain with direct or lateral pressure due to the keratoma.
2. Pain, plantar aspect of metatarsal on ambulation with or without foot gear.
3. Pain when walking barefoot on a hard floor.
4. May complain of dorsally located digits.
5. May complain of walking on a bone or pebble.
6. May complain of arthritis.

Preoperative X-ray Evaluation

1. Degenerative changes of metatarsal-phalangeal joint may be present.
2. Epiphysis of the metatarsal should be closed.
3. Prominent plantar condyle appears on axial X-ray.
4. Metatarsal head may appear depressed compared to adjacent metatarsals on the axial view.
5. Toe may appear dorsally contracted.
6. Hammertoe may be present.
7. Subluxation of the metatarsal-phalangeal joint may be present.

Biomechanical Evaluation

1. The procedure may be performed in the presence of uncontrollable pronatory forces.
2. Postoperative orthotic control should be utilized if necessary.

Surgical Procedure

A three to four centimeter curvilinear incision is made over the dorsal aspect of the metatarsal-phalangeal joint. By using sharp and blunt dissection, the extensor tendon is freed. It is usually necessary to perform a Z-lengthening in the extensor tendon, which may be performed at this time. The capsule of the metatarsal-phalangeal joint may now be visualized. A dorsal linear incision is made through the capsule. The head of the metatarsal is delivered into the wound by freeing the capsule and incising the collateral ligaments. The anterior one-third of the metatarsal head and the plantar portion of the head are excised with an osteotome and mallet. Care must be taken to remove the plantar condyles on the frontal plane and not leave a prominent shelf of bone. The cut surfaces are then rounded and smoothed with a rasp. The area is flushed well with sterile saline. The capsule is repaired with 3-0 or 4-0 absorbable sutures and the subcutaneous tissue is approximated to close any dead space. The skin may be approximated with 4-0 or 5-0 simple interrupted sutures or a running subcuticular type suture. The plantar lesion may be ellipsed if it appears well demarcated and fibrotic.

Postoperative Management

The patient is placed in a compression bandage and is allowed to ambulate within 24 hours in Bevin shoes. The sutures are removed at the end of 10 days to two weeks. At this time the postoperative X-rays may be taken. The patient may begin to return to regular foot gear in two to three weeks following surgery.

Advantages

1. May be performed on older people.
2. Minimal disability is expected following the procedure.
3. The eradication of the lesion, if it is due to a prominent condyle.

Disadvantages

1. Disruption of the integrity of the metatarsal-phalangeal joint is necessary.
2. Limitation of motion at the metatarsal-phalangeal joint is necessary.
2. Limitation of motion at the metatarsal-phalangeal joint may result.
3. No control is present over the height of the metatarsal.
4. Transfer lesions occur in a great many of the patients.
5. An uneven cut allows a portion of the metatarsal head to remain prominent.

The steps in performing a plantar condylectomy are illustrated. First the anterior portion of the metatarsal is remodeled, followed by resection of the plantar condyles. All sharp edges are then rounded and smoothed. The last diagram is a frontal view showing the correct plane to resect the condyles. It should be noted that the fibular condyle is larger and more prominent than the medial condyle.

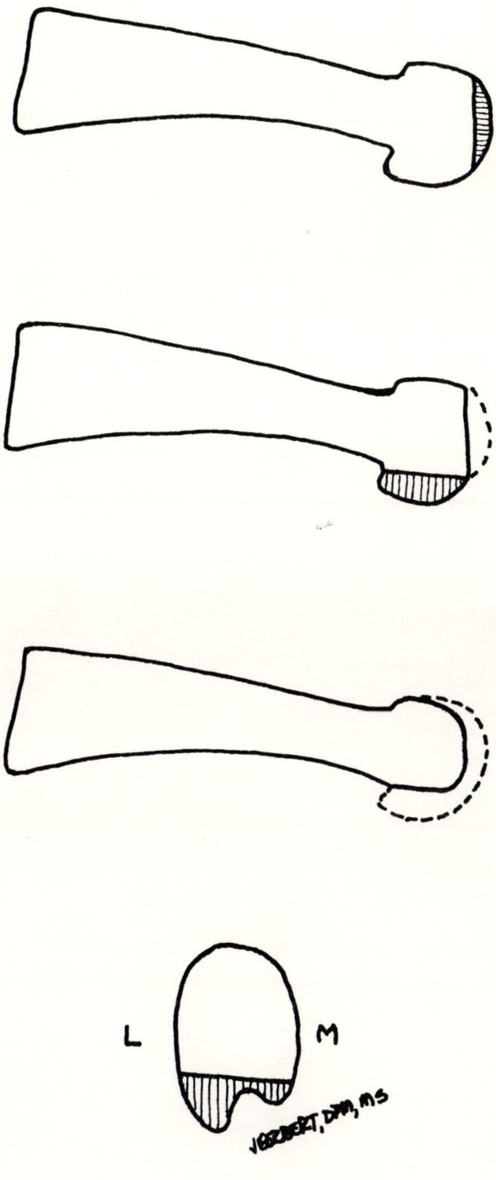

FIGURE 1
PLANTAR CONDYLECTOMY

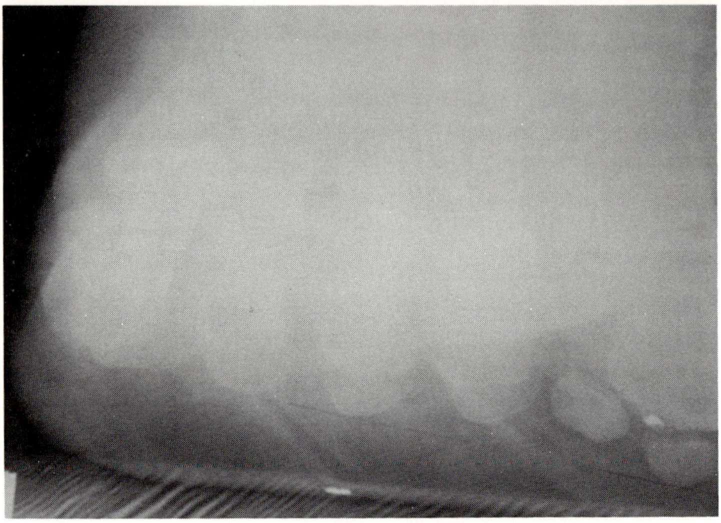

FIGURE 2A
PREOPERATIVE AXIAL X-RAY

Note the prominence of the head of the third metatarsal. Usually the shape of the head is round when visualized in this view. An intractable plantar keratoma was present under involved bone.

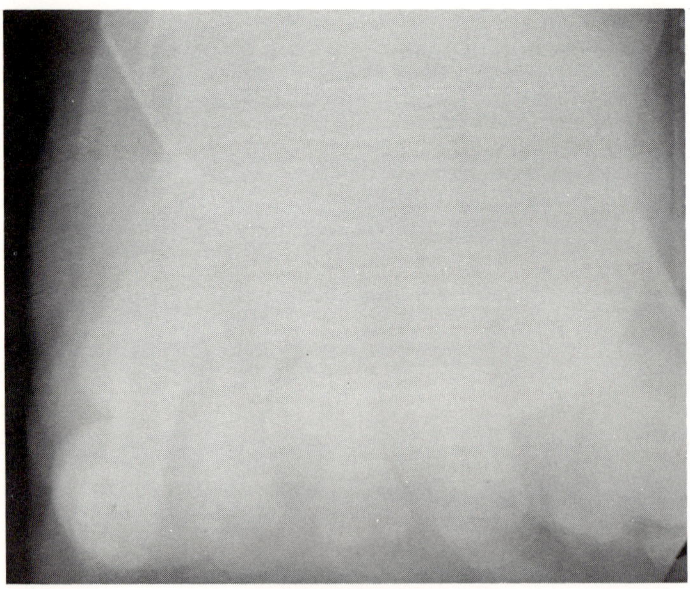

FIGURE 2B
POSTOPERATIVE AXIAL VIEW

On the postoperative axial view the plantar aspect of the third metatarsal is visualized. The cut was made so that more bone was removed from the fibular apsect of the head of the metatarsal.

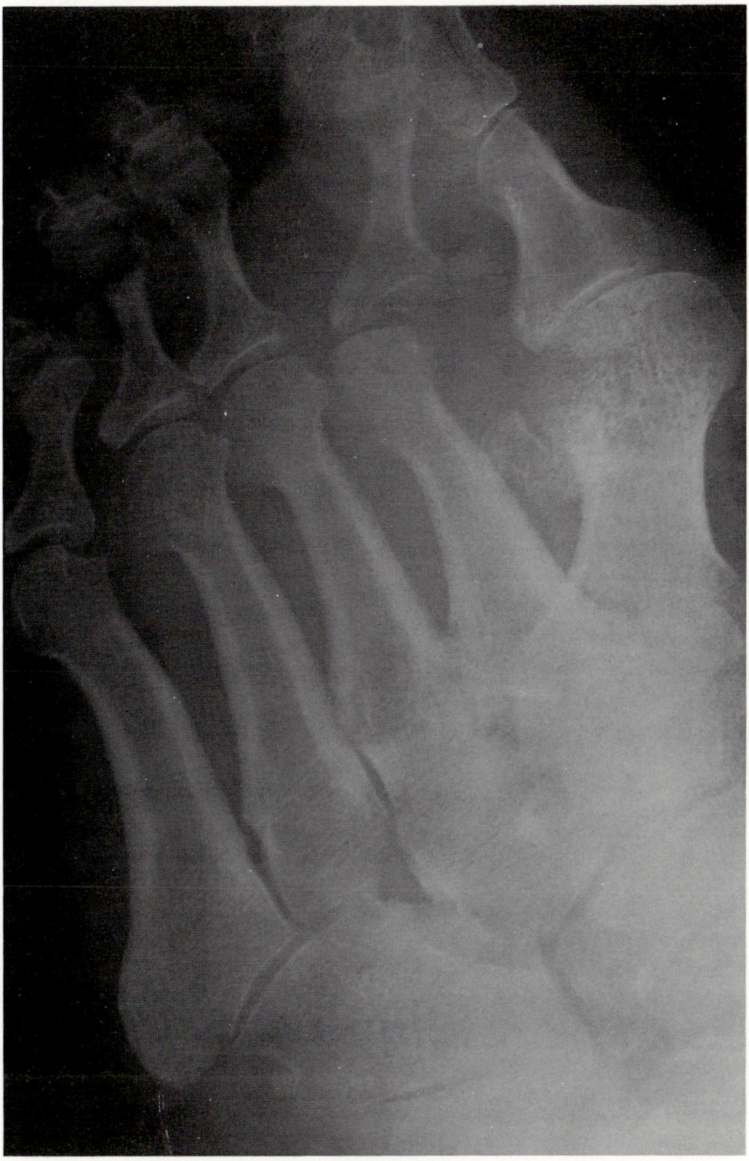

FIGURE 3
POSTOPERATIVE MEDIAL OBLIQUE X-RAY

A medial oblique view of the second metatarsal showing the postoperative appearance of the plantar condylectomy.

7. Metatarsal Head Resection

Preoperative Signs

1. Deformed metatarsal-phalangeal joint such as post Freibergs where the deformity is primarily at the metatarsal.
2. Articular disease of the metatarsal-phalangeal joint i.e. Rheumatoid arthritis.

Preoperative Symptoms

1. Pain on range of motion.
2. Dislocated or subluxed metatarsal-phalangeal joint as evidenced by digital dislocation.

Biomechanical Evaluation

1. Usually not significant in this procedure.
2. No consistent finding of biomechanical deformities.

Preoperative X-ray Evaluation

1. Diseased and deformed metatarsal-phalangeal joint.
2. The associated digit is dislocated or subluxed.
3. The affected metatarsal is excessively long.

Surgical Procedure

The approach for metatarsal head surgery in general is identical for the 2nd, 3rd and 4th metatarsals. The incision is placed lateral to the metatarsal-phalangeal joint and extends from mid-shaft of the proximal phalanx to mid-shaft of the metatarsal in a curvo-linear fashion. Subcutaneous tissue is then incised with care being taken to preserve the superficial veins and occasional digital nerves encountered. The next structure encountered is the long and short extensor tendons. These structures may be lengthened, sectioned or tenotomized depending on the type and extent of digital deformity present. The metatarsal-phalangeal joint capsule is next encountered and is usually entered via linear capsulotomy. All soft tissue capsular attachments are incised, the toe is plantarflexed, and the metatarsal head is delivered dorsally thru the wound. The surgical neck of the metatarsal is identified and the head resected using power equipment or hand equipment. Care must be exercised to remove slightly more plantar bone than dorsal. The cut is made straight across in the medial lateral direction.

Capsullorhapy is performed with an attempt being made to

hour-glass the capsule in the dead space. The incision is dressed with the associated digit held in correct position.

Occasionally, it may be necessary to place a K-wire through the toe and the metatarsal in an attempt to prevent digital retraction.

Postoperative Management

A postoperative shoe is dispensed, and weight-bearing is allowed 24 hours postoperative. Ambulation continues throughout, with suture removal 2 weeks postoperative. Return to shoes may be allowed in 2-4 weeks depending on edema and symptoms.

Advantages

1. Removal of diseased or deformed joints.

Disadvantages

1. Possible transfer lesion to adjacent metatarsal.
2. Digital retraction with the base of the proximal phalanx becoming the pathological agent.
3. Stump regeneration or degeneration.
4. Dorsally located digit.
5. Lesion reccurrence.

This represents a head resection of the lesser Metatarsals. The distal and plantar aspects are removed and remodeled.

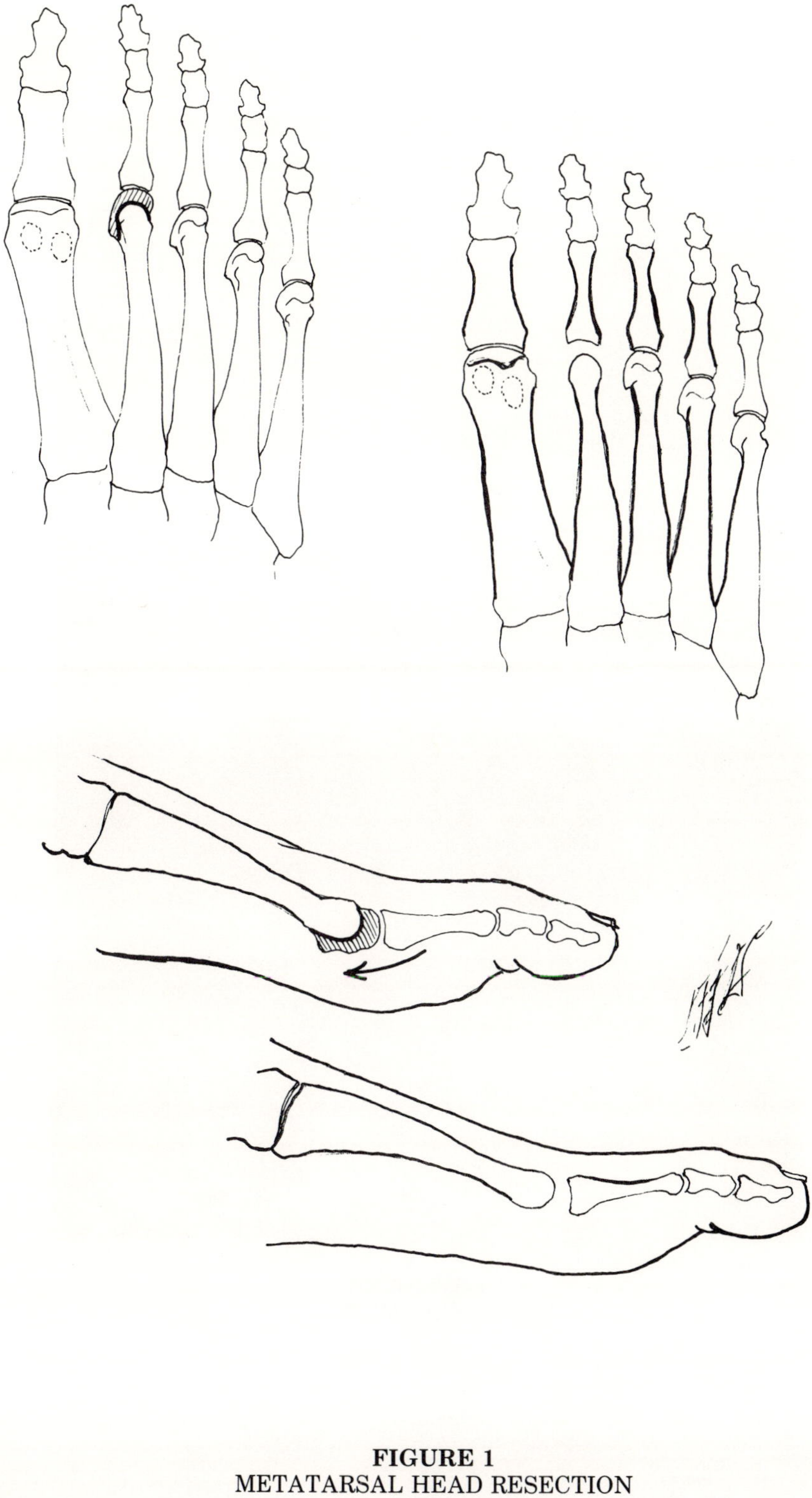

FIGURE 1
METATARSAL HEAD RESECTION

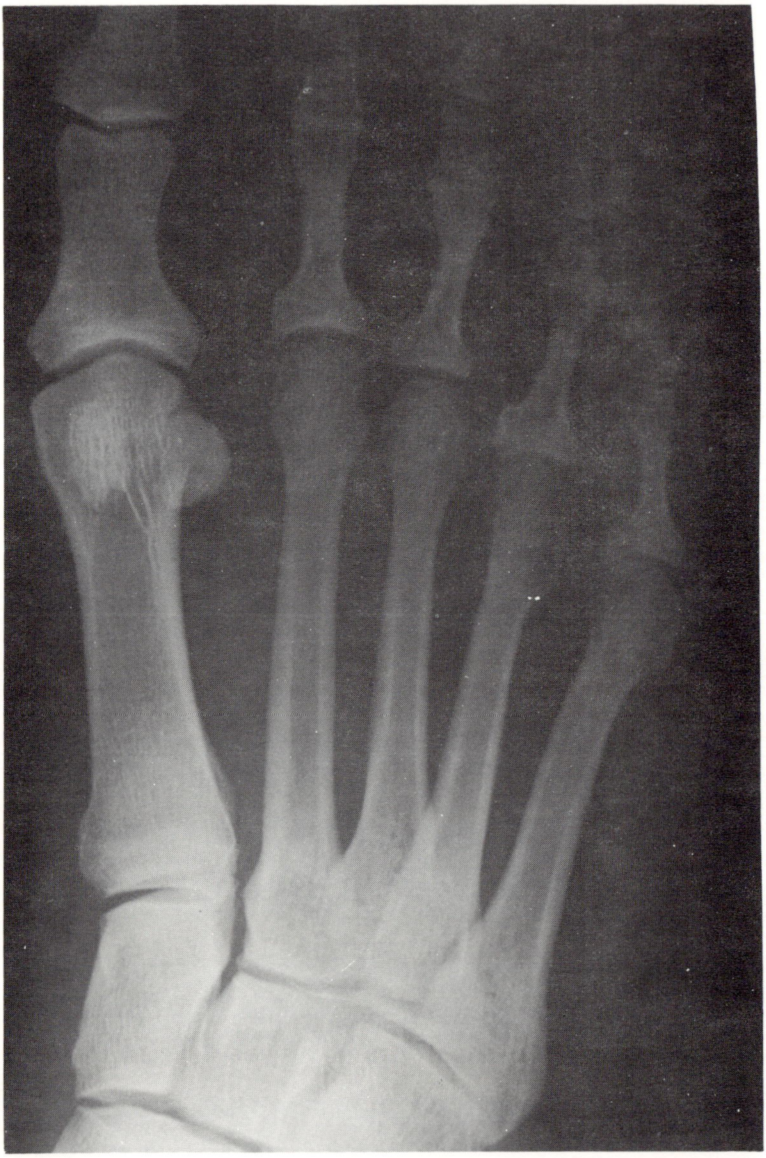

FIGURE 2A
PREOPERATIVE X-RAY

Note deformed fourth metatarsal head.

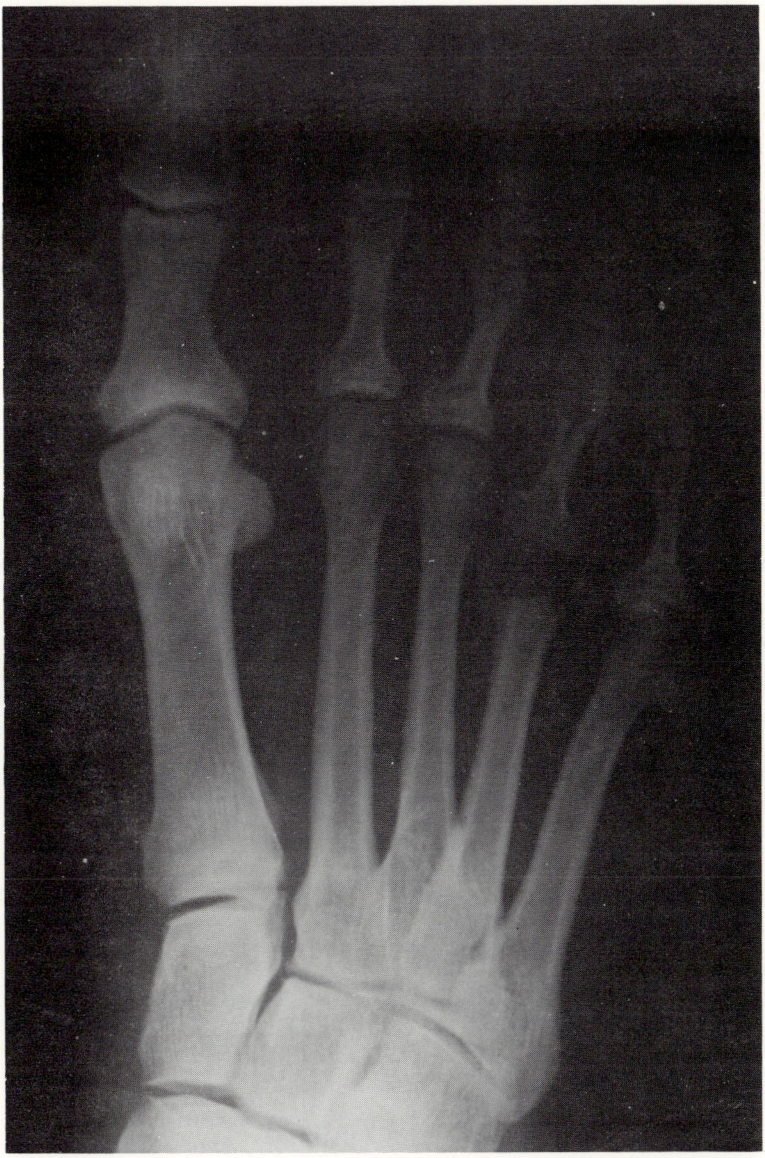

FIGURE 2B
POSTOPERATIVE X-RAY

This postoperative X-ray shows the deformed metatarsal head resected in toto.

Bibliography

Addante: Metatarsal osteotomy as a surgical approach for the elimination of Plantar Keratosis. *J.A.P.A.*, **8**:1969.

Borggrene, J.: Zur Operation Behandlung des Kontraken Spreiafusses. *Zeitsch. Orthop. Grenzb.*, **78**:581-582, 1949.

Billing, H. E.: Condylectomy for metatarsalgia: Indication and results. *Journal of the International College of Surgeons*, **25**:220, 1956.

Crenshaw, A. H.: *Cambell's Operative Orthopaedics, Vol. 2, 5th ed.*, C. V. Mosby, St. Louis, 1971, p. 1832.

DuVries, H. L.: New approach to the treatment of intractable verruca plantaris. *J.A.M.A.*, **152**:1202, 1953.

DuVries, H. L.: Verruca plantaris. *J.A.M.A.*, **154**:1302, 1954.

DuVries, H. L.: *Surgery of the Foot.* C. V. Mosby Company, St. Louis, 1973.

Giannestras, N. J.: Shortening of the metatarsal shaft for the correction of plantar keratosis. *Clin. Orthop.*, **4**:225, 1954.

Giannestras, N. J.: *Foot Disorders: Medical and Surgical Management.* Lea & Febiger, Philadelphia, 1973.

Jacoby, R.: V-osteoplasty for correction of intractable plantar keratosis. *J. Bone & Joint Surg.*, **49A**:61, 1958.

Kelikian, H.: *Hallux Valgus, Allied Deformities of the Forefoot and Metatarsalgia.* W. B. Saunders Co., Philadelphia, 1965.

Lowe, W. L.: *Metatarsal Head and Neck Osteotomies for Plantar Keratosis-1973.* Instructional Course at CCPM, Biomechanics Seminar, 1973.

Mau, C.: Eine Operation des Kontraken Spreizfusses. *Zol. Chir.*, **67**:667-670.

McKeever, D. C.: Operation for plantar callosities and metatarsalgia. *J. Bone & Joint Surg.*, **34A**:129, 1952.

Meisenbach, R. O.: Painful anterior arch of the foot: An operation for its relief by means of raising the arch. *Am. J. Ortho. Surg.*, **14**:206, 1916.

Rutherford, R.: Metatarsal shortening for the relief of symptomatic plantar keratosis. *J. Foot Surg.*, **9**:13, 1970.

Sgarlato, T. E.: *Compendium of Podiatric Biomechanics.* California College of Podiatric Medicine. San Francisco, 1971.

Drawings-Dorsal Wedge Osteotomy

S. Newell: *A Compendium of Podiatric Biomechanics.* California College of Podiatric Medicine, 1971, p. 413-420.

C. Fifth Metatarsal IPK

The intractable keratoma associated with the fifth metatarsal head may be located beneath the metatarsal head, lateral to the metatarsal head, or a combination of both types. Therefore one must carefully evaluate the lesion both from a clinical aspect and from a radiographic aspect in order to determine the exact etiology. This section of the monograph will deal with the various surgical procedures which can be employed depending upon the etiology of the lesion.

1. Closing Adductory Wedge Osteotomy of the Fifth Metatarsal

This procedure is a medial closing wedge osteotomy near the base of the fifth metatarsal. It is used for a situation where there is a lateral intractable keratoma at the fifth metatarsal head and where the fifth metatarsal-phalangeal joint is normal.

Preoperative Signs

1. A lateral keratoma in the area of the fifth metatarsal head.
2. A prominent fifth metatarsal laterally, especially on weight bearing.
3. A short fifth toe may be present.
4. The range of motion of the fifth metatarsal-phalangeal joint should be adequate and pain free.
5. Palpation between the fourth and fifth metatarsal heads reveals an abnormal separation.

Preoperative Symptoms

1. Pain around the fifth metatarsal head when wearing most types of foot gear.

2. Pain with direct pressure to lesion.
3. No complaint of discomfort when ambulating without shoes.
4. Patient many times complains of inability to wear many types of shoes due to wideness of foot.
5. No pain when fifth metatarsal-phalangeal joint is taken through its normal range of motion.

Preoperative X-ray Evaluation

1. Fifth metatarsal-phalangeal joint is within normal limits showing no degenerative changes.
2. The fifth metatarsal head is normal with no lateral condyle enlargement.
3. Definite bowing of fifth metatarsal and/or splaying of fifth metatarsal as compared to the fourth.
4. Abnormal intermetatarsal angle between fourth metatarsal and fifth.
5. Fifth metatarsal may be abnormally short.
6. Epiphysis may be open on fifth metatarsal.
7. Fifth metatarsal should be of normal bone density.

Biomechanical Evaluation

1. This procedure can be performed in the presence of uncontrollable pronatory forces.
2. Orthotic control should be instituted postoperatively if deemed necessary by the preoperative biomechnical evaluation.

Surgical Procedure

A five centimeter dorsolinear incision is made over the shaft and base of the fifth metatarsal just lateral to the extensor tendon. By use of sharp and blunt dissection the extensor tendon is exposed and retracted medially. The medial and lateral bounderies of the metatarsal shaft are palpated and a dorsolinear incision is made directly through the soft tissue and periosteum down to bone. The middle of this incision should be where the fourth metatarsal contacts the fifth. Using a sharp periosteal elevator the soft tissue and periosteum is freed from the dorsal and medial aspects of the metatarsal. A small amount is also freed from the lateral aspect of the bone. Score the amount of wedge to be excised from the fifth metatarsal where the fourth contacts it. Every attempt is made to perform the osteotomy as far proximal on the metatarsal as possible. The amount of bone to be removed can be calculated as in a closing or opening wedge osteotomy performed on the first metatarsal. This was described in detail in the first monograph of this series of Hallux Valgus. A 2 to 3 mm. wedge of bone usually suffices. By retracting from within the soft tissue - periosteal flap which has been freed from the bone, trauma to the neurovascular bundle in the fourth interspace can easily be avoided. Silk sutures can be inserted into this soft tissue-periosteal flap in order to easily identify it for closure after fixation of the osteotomy site. Attention is then directed toward the medial aspect of the bone where the osteotomy is started using either a reciprocating saber saw blade or a small, oscillating blade on a power hand piece. The cut is directed perpendicular to the long axis of the shaft of the metatarsal. This is extremely important while performing a uni-plane osteotomy if one does not want the metatarsal to move in either a dorsiflexed or plantarflexed position at the time the osteotomy site is closed. While performing the osteotomy care is taken to preserve the lateral cortex of the bone. Once the desired amount of bone wedge is excised the site is closed by applying pressure distally while stabilizing the proximal segment. The site should be closed without undue tension on the lateral cortex. The entire surgical site should be flushed with copious amounts of sterile saline. Fixation of the osteotomy site is best accomplished by use of 28 gauge monofilament stainless steel wire. The method for securing the wire fixation varies depending upon the surgeon's preference. When the osteotomy has been performed as far proximal on the fifth metatarsal as possible then fixation should be as follows: Depending upon the size of the fifth metatarsal, place 1 or 2 drill holes dorso-medial and dorsal distal to the osteotomy site and angulated into the site. Proximal to the osteotomy site place 1 or 2 drill holes depending upon the size of the bone angulated into the osteotomy site. The wire is threaded through the drill holes and twisted as described for the first metatarsal osteotomy procedure. If you wish to use a horizontal wire fixation of the osteotomy then the osteotomy site must be made just distal to where the fourth metatarsal contacts the fifth. This is necessary in order to retrieve the proximal wire for fixation. The wire is threaded through two horizontal drill holes, one on either side of the osteotomy site, extending from lateral to medial with the wire being tied on the medial aspect of the shaft. After the wire has been twisted down to close the osteotomy site it is cut in such a manner as to leave a small tag which can be inserted into one of the drill holes. The soft tissue-periosteal flap is approximated over the osteotomy site using 4-0 or 5-0 absorbable sutures. The subcutaneous tissue is closed to obliterate any dead space. The skin is approximated using either a 5-0 nylon simple interrupted suture or a subcuticular closure.

Postoperative Management

The patient is placed in a below-the-knee cast with a walker and ambulation is instituted within 24 to 36 hours following surgery. If performed in a hospital, the average hospital stay has been 3 days. The cast is changed approximately 3 weeks postoperatively and the sutures removed. X-rays are also taken at this time. Another below-the-knee cast with a walker is applied for an additional 3 weeks. Clinical findings and X-ray evaluation are used to determine the duration of cast immobilization. Following cast removal the usual physical therapy is instituted and biomechanical control is initiated if needed. In summary one can state that the postoperative management of the patient is very similar to the management of a patient with a fracture of the fifth metatarsal. It should also be stated that the majority of patients return to their regular footgear in 7 to 8 weeks following surgery.

Advantages

1. Preserves the fifth metatarsal-phalangeal joint.
2. Can be performed on a short fifth ray.
3. Corrects a deformity within the shaft of the fifth metatarsal.
4. Can be performed in young patients where the epiphyseal area is open.
5. Does not alter the dorsi-plantar position of the fifth ray if performed properly.

Disadvantages

1. Due to the pyramiding of the bases of the metatarsals it is difficult to perform the osteotomy in cancellous bone which therefore results in delayed bony healing at times.
2. Disruption of the internal fixation along with improper immobilization could result in a poor alignment of the metatarsal.
3. Immobilization in plaster is usually required for 6 weeks.
4. Prolonged disability as compared to fifth metatarsal head resection.
5. Does not correct a plantar intractable keratoma.

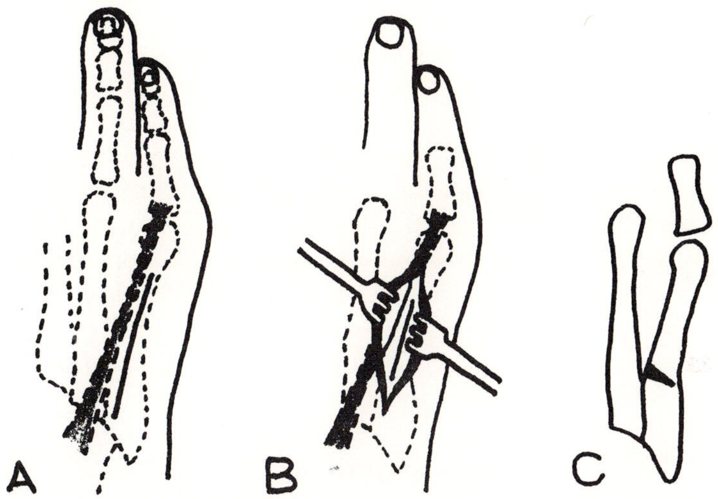

FIGURE 1
CLOSING ADDUCTORY WEDGE OSTEOTOMY

A. A dorsal linear incision is made just lateral to the extensor digitorum longus tendon and over the shaft of the fifth metatarsal.

B. Adequate exposure is obtained through this type of incision and the tendon is retracted medially. A dorsal linear incision is then made directly over the proximal aspect of the fifth metatarsal through soft tissue and periosteum.

C. The osteotomy site is made approximately at the level where the fourth metatarsal contacts the fifth metatarsal. The shaded area represents the osseous wedge to be removed which is usually 2 to 3 millimeters.

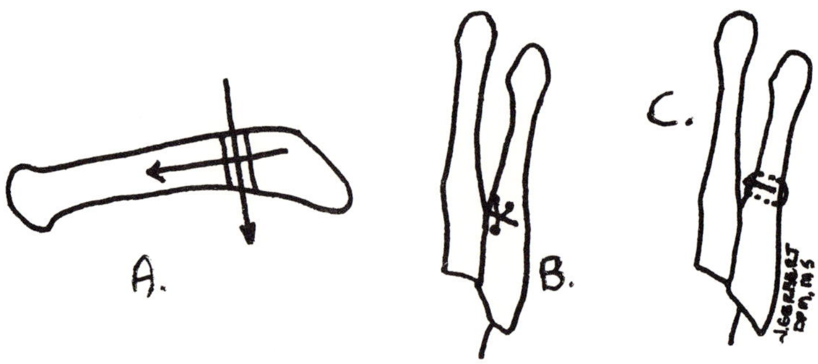

FIGURE 2

CLOSING ADDUCTORY WEDGE OSTEOTOMY

A. This view shows the metatarsal from medial with the wedge removed. Note how the angulation of the cut is from dorsal-distal to plantar-proximal which is perpendicular to the long axis of the metatarsal shaft.

B. This view shows the osteotomy site closed. The fixation was obtained by drilling two holes distal to the osteotomy site and one proximal.

C. This view shows another way in which the osteotomy site may be closed using a horizontal-type stainless steel wire fixation. Two drill holes are made, one on either side of the osteotomy site, extending from lateral to medial. Note how in this case the osteotomy site must be made more distal to where the fourth metatarsal contacts the fifth in order to technically use a horizontal wire fixation.

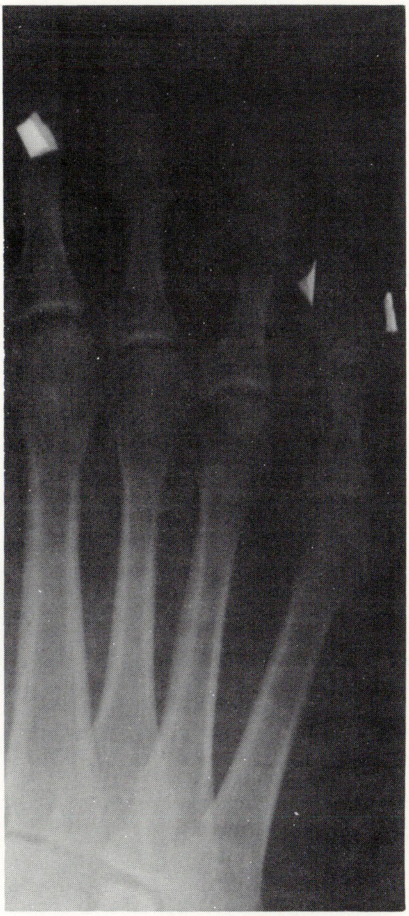

FIGURE 3A
PREOPERATIVE A-P X-RAY

Note the splaying of the fifth metatarsal. Clinically, the patient had a lateral hyperkeratotic lesion over the fifth metatarsal head area.

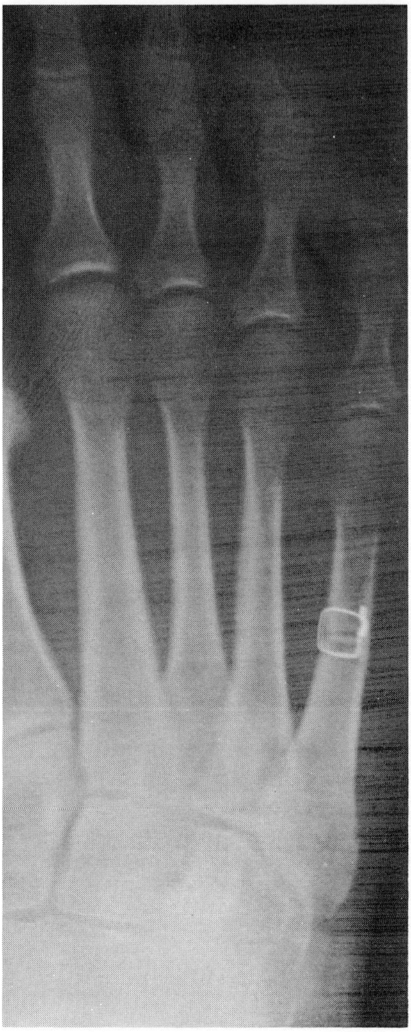

FIGURE 3B
POSTOPERATIVE A-P X-RAY

Following closing adductory wedge osteotomy of the fifth metatarsal. Fixation was accomplished using a horizontal mattress suture of 28 gauge monofilament stainless steel wire. Note how the lateral cortex was left intact. The osteotomy should be performed in the midshaft of the metatarsal, as shown here, if at all possible, in order to achieve better and faster healing.

2. Dorsal Wedge Osteotomy

This procedure is a dorsal osteotomy performed as far proximal on the metatarsal as technically possible. It is used for the situation where there is a plantar intractable keratoma at the fifth metatarsal head secondary to a depressed fifth metatarsal.

Preoperative Signs

1. A plantar intractable keratoma is present in the area of the fifth metatarsal head.
2. The fifth metatarsal head is prominent when palpated plantarly as compared to the other metatarsal heads.
3. The dorsal aspect of the fifth metatarsal head is not prominent upon weight bearing.
4. A short fifth toe may be present.
5. The range of motion of the fifth metatarsal-phalangeal joint is adequate and pain free.
6. Fifth toe may be dorsally contracted at the metatarsophalangeal joint.

Preoperative Symptoms

1. Pain around the fifth metatarsal head when wearing most type of foot gear.
2. Pain upon direct pressure to the plantar lesion.
3. The patient may complain of discomfort when ambulating without shoes.
4. No pain when the fifth metatarsal-phalangeal joint is taken through its normal range of motion.

Biomechanical Evaluation

1. A forefoot varus deformity is a very common finding.
2. This procedure can be performed in the presence of uncontrollable pronatory forces.
3. Orthotic control should be instituted postoperatively if deemed necessary by the preoperative biomechanical exam.

Preoperative X-ray Evaluation

1. Fifth metatarsal-phalangeal joint is within normal limits showing no degenerative changes.
2. The fifth metatarsal head is within normal limits.
3. Fifth toe may appear abnormally short.
4. Epiphysis may be open on fifth metatarsal.
5. Fifth metatarsal should be of normal bone density.

6. Fifth metatarsal head appears depressed as seen on an axial view of the foot.
7. Fifth toe may appear dorsally contracted.

Surgical Procedure

A three to four cm. dorsolinear incision is made over the proximal aspect of the metatarsal shaft and base area just lateral to the extensor digitorum longus tendon. By use of sharp and blunt dissection, the extensor tendon is exposed and retracted medially. The medial and lateral bounderies of the metatarsal shaft are palpated and a dorsolinear incision is made through the overlying soft tissue and periosteum. The middle of this incision should be where the fourth metatarsal contacts the fifth. Using a sharp periosteal elevator the soft tissue and periosteum is freed from the dorsal-medial and dorsal-lateral aspects of the metatarsal to expose the area of bone to be excised. Every attempt is made to perform the osteotomy as far proximal on the metatarsal as technically possible in order to promote better osseous healing. However going further proximal than where the fourth metatarsal contacts the fifth will present problems with the flare of the metatarsal as the styloid process begins to take form. The amount of bone to be excised can be calculated preoperatively as described for the dorsal wedge of the first metatarsal. Usually 2 millimeters of bone is sufficient for correction. The osteotomy is best performed by using a small oscillating blade on a power hand piece. Care is taken not to cut completely through the bone but rather leave the plantar cortex intact. One should keep in mind that the fifth metatarsal is not a square bone but rather triangular in shape. Therefore a good way to prevent cutting completely through the bone is to keep checking for the medullary canal and use the floor of the canal as an indication of the proximity of the plantar cortex. The proximal cut is made perpendicular to the long axis of the metatarsal shaft. The distal cut is angled proximal to meet the first cut. The area should be flushed with copious amounts of sterile saline. Once the desired amount of bone has been excised the osteotomy site can be closed by either using one drill hole proximal and one distal or, if the bone is large enough, two drill holes distally. The drill holes should be angled into the osteotomy site. The fixation is accomplished using 28 gauge monofilament stainless steel wire threaded through the holes and twisted down as described for the osteotomy on the first metatarsal. Closure of the osteotomy site before twisting the wire should be without undue tension on the plantar cortex. The soft tissue-periosteal flaps are approximated using 4-0 or 5-0 absorbable sutures. The subcutaneous tissue is approximated to close any dead space. The skin is approximated using either 4-0 or 5-0 nylon simple interrupted sutures or a running subcuticular suture. You can clinically ascertain whether the metatarsal has been dorsiflexed sufficiently by examining the plantar skin under the fifth metatarsal head. A small amount of dimpling should be seen, which indicates the metatarsal head has been dorsiflexed. At this time the plantar intractable lesion should be ellipsed if it appears well demarcated and fibrotic.

Postoperative Management

The patient is placed in a below-the-knee plaster cast with a walker and ambulation is instituted within 24 to 36 hours postoperatively. If performed in the hospital, the average hospital stay has been 3 days. The cast is changed in three weeks and the sutures are removed. X-rays are taken at this time and another below-the-knee walking cast is applied. This cast is maintained for an additional three weeks. Following cast removal the usual physical therapy is instituted and biomechanical therapy is initiated if needed. The patient can usually return to regular foot gear in 7 to 8 weeks following surgery.

Advantages

1. Preserves the fifth metatarsal-phalangeal joint.
2. Can be performed in the presence of a short fifth toe.
3. Can be performed in young patients with an open epiphysis.
4. May help to reduce a dorsally contracted fifth toe.
5. Can be performed with a minimal amount of soft tissue dissection.

Disadvantages

1. Does not correct a lateral keratotic lesion at the fifth metatarsal head area.
2. Prolonged disability as compared to a fifth metatarsal head resection.
3. Immobilization in plaster for approximately six weeks.
4. Disruption of the internal fixation along with improper immobilization could result in poor alignment of the bone.
5. Due to the pyramiding of the bases of the metatarsals it is difficult to perform the osteotomy in cancellous bone which therefore results in delayed osseous healing at times.
6. Removal of too much bone can result in a dorsiflexed metatarsal which is non-weight bearing and produces limitation of motion at the metatarsal-phalangeal joint.

A. This diagram shows the pyramiding of the base of the fourth metatarsal to the fifth and the approximate area where the osteotomy will have to be performed.

B. This is a dorsal view of the metatarsal showing the bone to be excised.

C. This is a lateral or medial view of the metatarsal showing the amount of bone to be excised. Note that the plantar cortex is kept intact.

D. This is a lateral or medial view showing the osteotomy site closed and the new position of the metatarsal head. The metatarsal is dorsiflexed and shortened to slight extent.

E. This is a lateral or medial view showing the dorsal drill holes being made which are angulated into the osteotomy site.

F. This is a dorsal view showing the three drill holes made for fixation. If the metatarsal is small in width one drill hole on either side of the osteotomy site may be used in place of two distally.

G. This is a dorsal view showing the stainless steel wire threaded through the drill holes.

H. This dorsal view demonstrates the wire being twisted down to close and secure the osteotomy site.

I. This dorsal view shows the osteotomy site closed and the wire cut and reinserted into one of the drill holes.

J. This is a frontal plane view of the forefoot (axial view type) showing a plantar depressed fifth metatarsal.

K. This frontal plane view shows the metatarsal heads in good alignment after a dorsal wedge osteotomy of the fifth metatarsal.

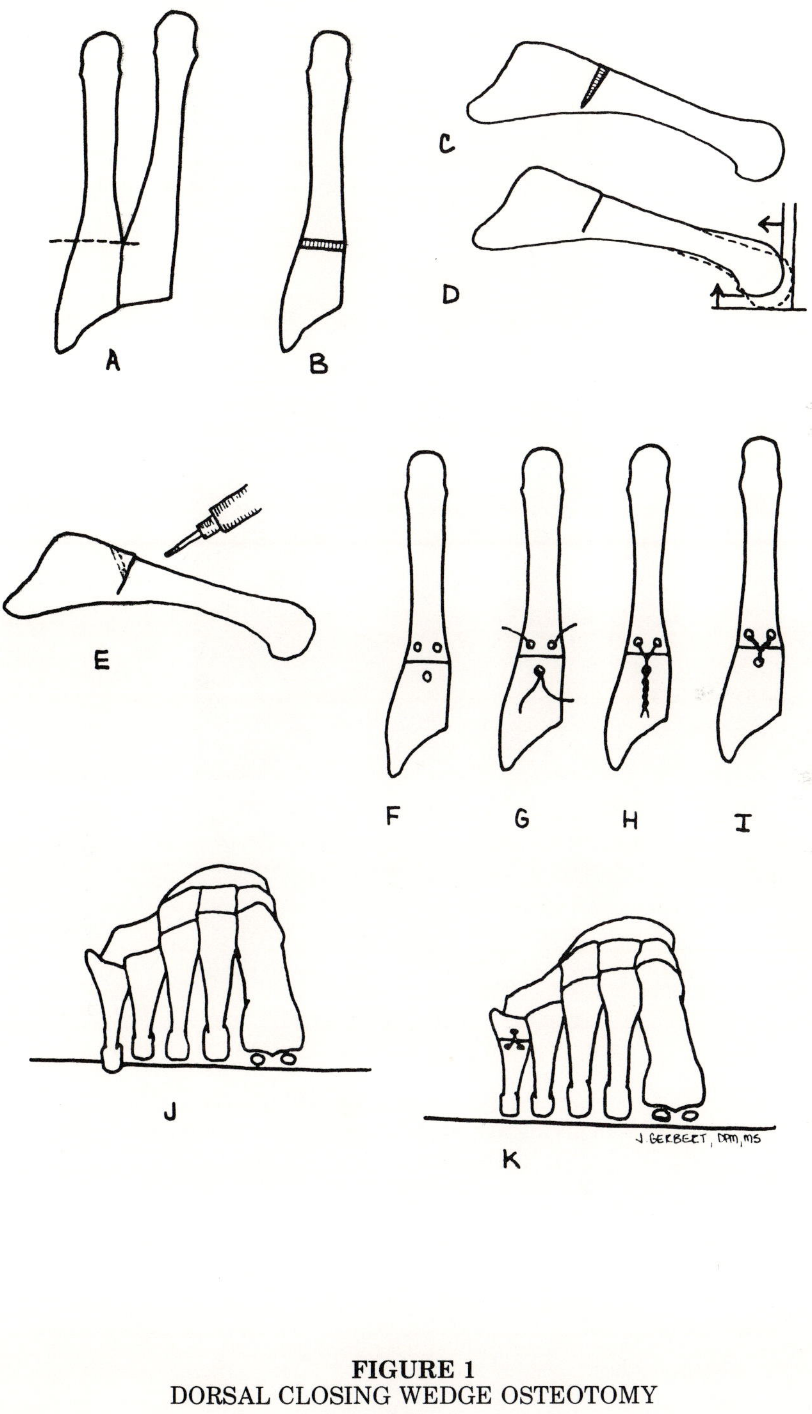

FIGURE 1
DORSAL CLOSING WEDGE OSTEOTOMY

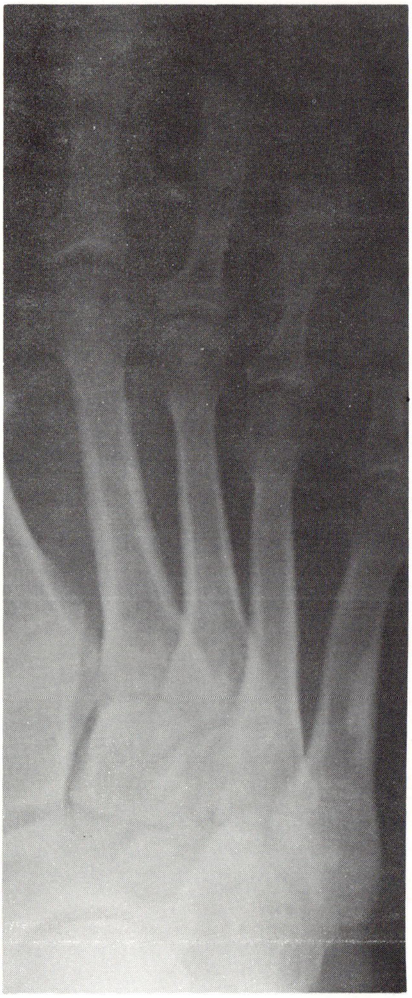

FIGURE 2A
PREOPERATIVE A-P X-RAY

Note the mild abductory deviation occurring at the metatarsal neck. However, this patient had a hyperkeratotic plantar lesion directly under the fifth metatarsal head.

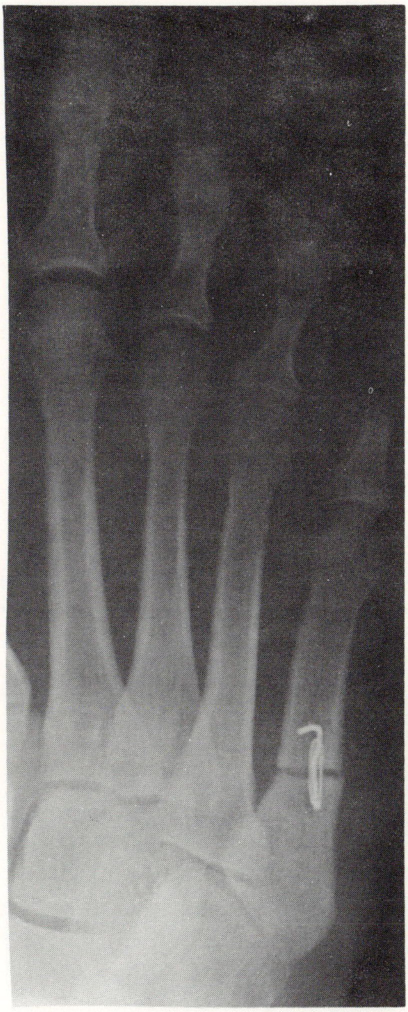

FIGURE 2B
POSTOPERATIVE A-P X-RAY

Following a dorsal closing wedge osteotomy of the fifth metatarsal. Some adduction of the metatarsal occurred due to the angulation of the osteotomy cut from dorsal to plantar. Fixation was accomplished using 28 gauge monofilament stainless steel wire.

3. Bi-Plane Osteotomy of the Fifth Metatarsal

This procedure is a combination of the medial closing wedge osteotomy and the dorsal closing wedge osteotomy. It is used for the situation where there is a plantar and lateral intractable keratoma at the fifth metatarsal head and one wishes to preserve the fifth metatarsal-phalangeal joint.

Preoperative Signs

1. A plantar and lateral intractable keratoma is present in the area of the fifth metatarsal head.
2. The dorsal aspect of the fifth metatarsal head is not prominent upon weight bearing.
3. A short fifth toe may be present.
4. The range of motion of the fifth metatarsal-phalangeal joint must be adequate and free of pain.
5. Palpation between the fourth and fifth metatarsal heads reveals an abnormal separation.
6. Fifth metatarsal head is prominent when palpated plantarly as compared to the other metatarsal heads.

Preoperative Symptoms

1. Pain around the fifth metatarsal head when wearing most type of foot gear.
2. Pain with direct pressure to the lesions.
3. The patient may complain of discomfort in the involved area when ambulating without shoes.
4. The patient many times complains of the inability to wear many types of shoes due to the wideness of the foot.
5. No pain when the fifth metatarsal-phalangeal joint is taken through its normal range of motion.

Biomechanical Evaluation

1. A forefoot varus deformity is a very common finding.
2. This procedure can be performed in the presence of uncontrollable pronatory forces.
3. Orthotic control should be instituted postoperatively if deemed necessary by the preoperative biomechanical exam.

Preoperative X-ray Evaluation

1. Fifth metatarsal-phalangeal joint is within normal limits showing no degenerative changes.
2. The first metatarsal head is normal with no lateral condyle enlargement.
3. Definite bowing of the fifth metatarsal and/or splaying of the fifth metatarsal as compared to the fourth.

4. Abnormal intermetatarsal angle between the fourth and fifth metatarsals.
5. Fifth ray may be abnormally short.
6. Epiphysis may be open of fifth metatarsal.
7. Fifth metatarsal should be of normal bone density.
8. Fifth metatarsal is depressed as seen on an axial view of the foot.

Surgical Procedure

A 5 cm dorsolinear incision is made over the shaft and base of the fifth metatarsal just lateral to the extensor tendon. By use of sharp and blunt dissection the extensor tendon is exposed and retracted medially. The medial and lateral bounderies of the metatarsal shaft are palpated and a dorsolinear incision is made directly through the soft tissue and periosteum down to bone. The middle of this incision should be where the fourth metatarsal contacts the fifth. Using a sharp periosteal elevator the soft tissue and periosteum is freed from the dorsal, medial, and dorsal-lateral aspects of the shaft. The amount of wedge to be excised from the fifth metatarsal is scored where the fourth metatarsal contacts it. Every attempt is made to perform the osteotomy as far proximal on the metatarsal as possible. Since there is no accurate way at this time to determine preoperatively the amount of bone to be removed in making a bi-plane osteotomy, it has been found that a wedge of 2 to 3 millimeters usually suffices. By retracting from within the soft tissue-periosteal flap which has been freed from the metatarsal shaft both medially and laterally trauma to the neurovascular bundle in the fourth interspace can easily be avoided. Attention is then directed toward the medial aspect of the bone where the osteotomy is started using either a reciprocating saber blade or a small oscillating blade on a power hand piece. The most proximal cut is made perpendicular to the long axis of the shaft of the metatarsal. The distal cut is angled from dorsal-distal to plantar-proximal in order to achieve the dorsiflexed position of the head of the metatarsal when the osteotomy is closed. In the uni-plane medial closing wedge osteotomy the lateral cortex was kept intact; however in the bi-plane osteotomy the only portion of the cortex which remains intact is the plantar-lateral aspect. Therefore extreme care must be used when excising the wedge of bone so as not to cut completely through the metatarsal at this plantar-lateral aspect. Once the desired amount of bone is excised the site is closed by applying pressure distally in a dorsiflexory and adductory manner while stabilizing the proximal segment. The area should be flushed with copious amounts of sterile saline. Fixation is best accomplished using 28 gauge monofiliment stainless steel wire. This type of osteotomy is closed by placing two drill holes distal to the osteotomy site and one proximal to the site. The holes distally are dorso-medial and dorsal and the hole proximal is dorsal. The drill holes are made far enough from the osteotomy site in order not to fracture through the osteotomy site and are angled into the site at the level of the medullary canal. The wire is threaded through the drill holes and twisted down, closing the osteotomy site as described for the first metatarsal osteotomy. The soft tissue-periosteal flaps are approximated over the osteotomy site using 4-0 or 5-0 absorbable sutures. The subcutaneous tissue is closed to obliterate any dead space. The skin is approximated using either a 5-0 nylon simple interrupted closure or a subcuticular closure. The plantar lesion can be ellipsed if desired.

Postoperative Management

The patient is placed in a below-the-knee cast with a walker and ambulation is instituted within 24 to 36 hours following surgery. If patient is hospitalized, the average hospital stay is 3 days. The cast is changed three weeks postoperatively and the sutures removed. X-rays are taken at this time to determine if alignment is good and how healing is progressing. Another below-the-knee cast with a walker is applied for an additional three weeks. X-rays are once again taken to evaluate the healing process and whether plaster immobilization can be discontinued. Following cast removal the usual physical therapy is instituted and biomechanical control is initiated if needed. The majority of patients can return to their regular footgear in 8 to 10 weeks following surgery.

Advantages

1. The fifth metatarsal-phalangeal joint is preserved.
2. This procedure can be performed on a short fifth ray.
3. Corrects a deformity of the metatarsal shaft itself.
4. Can be performed in young patients where the epiphyseal area is open.
5. Corrects both a plantar and lateral intractable lesion at the same time.

Disadvantages

1. Hospitalization is usually required for the patient.
2. Due to the pyramiding of the bases of the metatarsals it is difficult to perform the osteotomy in cancellous bone which therefore results in delayed bone healing to some extent.

4. Disruption of the internal fixation along with improper immobilization could result in a poor alignment of the metatarsal.
5. Immobilization in a plaster cast is usually required for six weeks.
6. Prolonged disability as compared to a fifth metatarsal head resection or condylectomy.
7. Requires advanced surgical skills in order to excise a bone wedge on two planes and leave a certain amount of cortex intact.

A. This drawing shows a cross-section through the shaft of the metatarsal and the extent of the plantar-lateral cortex which remains intact.

B. This view of the medial aspect of the metatarsal demonstrates the difference in the angulation of the cuts in removing the wedge from the bone.

C. This is a dorsal view showing the wedge of bone removed and the drill holes placed distal and proximal to the osteotomy site for the purpose of fixation. Note how the only intact portion of bone is the plantar lateral aspect.

D. This is a dorsal view demonstrating the closure of the osteotomy site using stainless steel wire.

E. These two illustrations show the three dimensional aspect of the bi-plane osteotomy. The stippled area in each drawing represents the intact portion of the lateral cortex after the osteotomy site is completed.

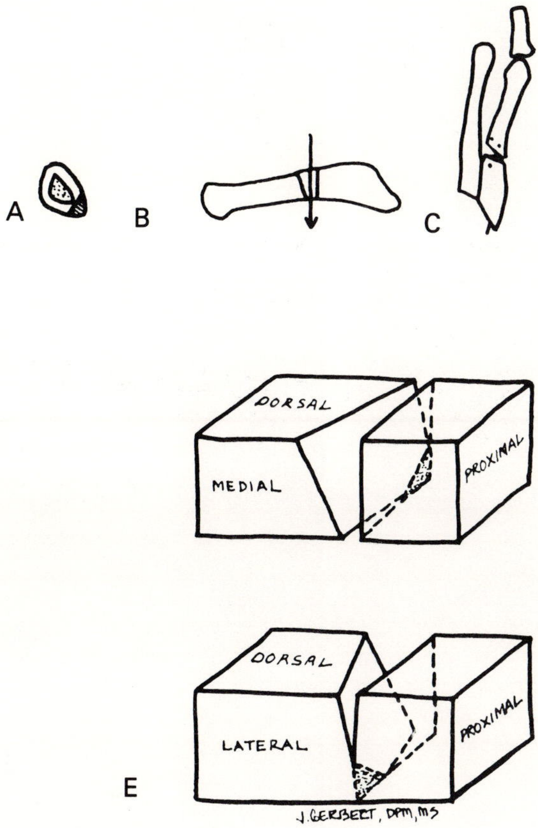

FIGURE 1
BIPLANE OSTEOTOMY

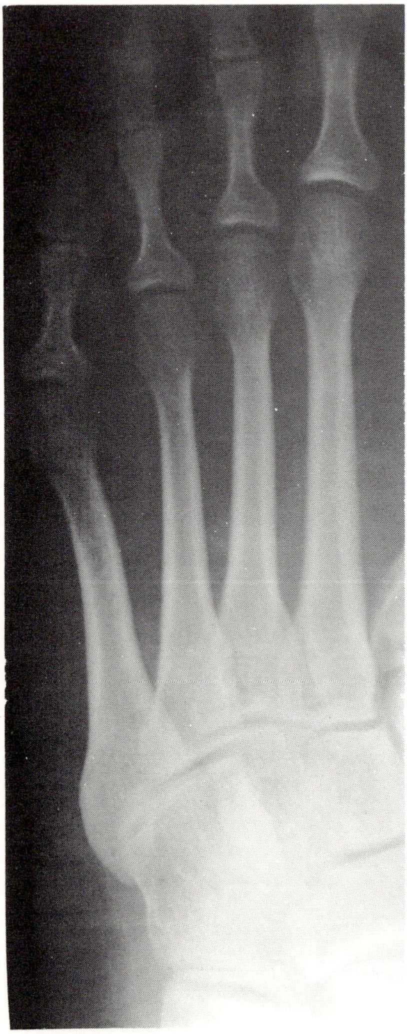

FIGURE 2A
PREOPERATIVE A-P X-RAY

Note splaying of the fifth metatarsal. Clinically, the metatarsal was also depressed. The patient had a plantar and lateral hyperkeratotic lesion.

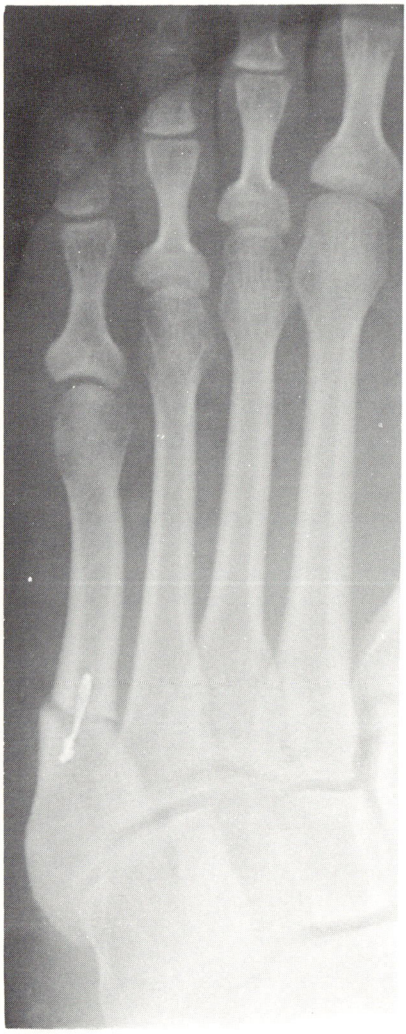

FIGURE 2B
POSTOPERATIVE A-P X-RAY

This is a non-weight bearing A-P X-ray postoperative following a biplane osteotomy of the fifth metatarsal. The metatarsal was raised dorsally and adducted. Fixation was accomplished by use of a double strand of 28 gauge monofilament stainless steel wire.

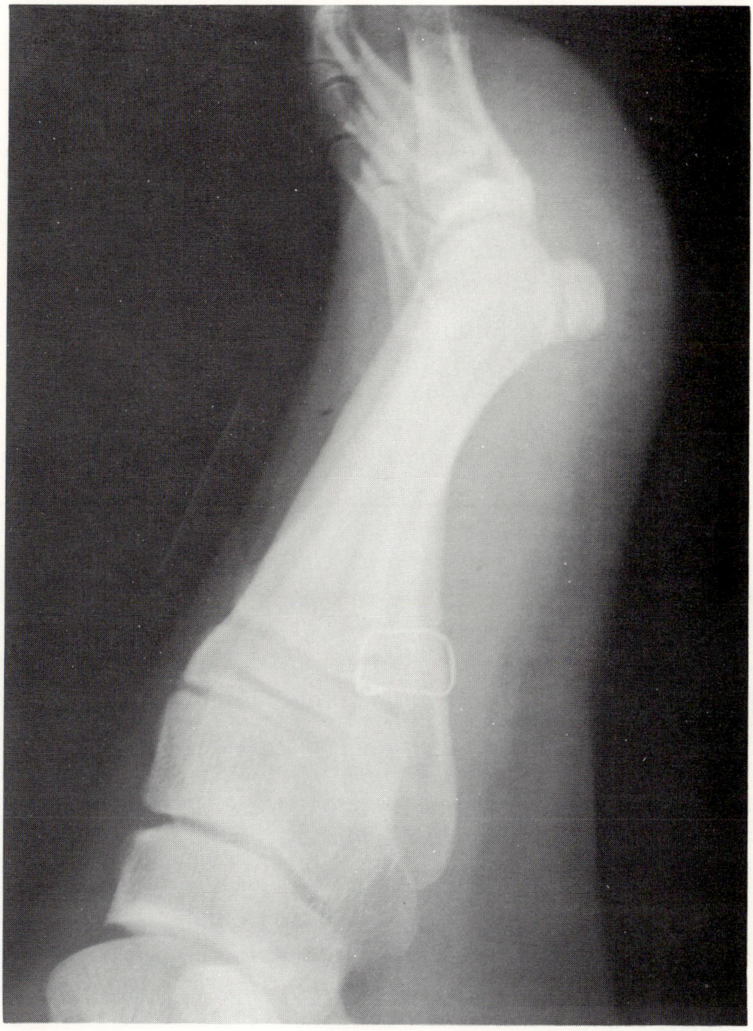

FIGURE 3
POSTOPERATIVE M-O X-RAY

This is an M-O view which demonstrates the fixation of the biplane osteotomy dorsal to plantar through the metatarsal.

4. Osteoclasis-type Procedure

(Open Metaphyseal Osteotomy)

The open metaphyseal osteotomy is presented as a surgical technique for the treatment of the intractible plantar keratoma beneath the head of the fifth metatarsal. This technique is essentially the same as the open metaphyseal osteotomy for treatment of intractable plantar keratoma beneath the second, third, and fourth metatarsal heads except modifications are made in the surgical technique and post-surgical padding and bandaging. This technique also maintains the basic forefoot architecture and allows retrograde forces incurred during ambulation to dorsiflex and adduct the surgically freed metatarsal head to its proper level and attitude to the midline of the foot. Shearing forces beneath the fifth metatarsal head are minimized and transferred more evenly across the forefoot as the metatarsal moves dorsally. Ambulation is allowed immediately following surgery if done in the office, or the following day if in the hospital. Long postoperative care periods are not necessary and patients need not be burdened with casts, long periods of immobilization and medications.

The surgical technique described in this chapter is performed using the Lombodi osteotome and Rush mallet. However, other bone cutting instruments may also be used, such as the bone cutter or power instruments such as the Stryker reciprocating bone saw, Hall, Ritter and other power instruments using burrs such as the Lindnear, Probber or Shannon burrs. Minimal surgical dissection is the key to success in this procedure which has achieved good to excellent results in over 80% of the patients upon whom open metaphyseal osteotomy was performed to cause the resolution of intractable plantar keratomas.

Preoperative Signs

1. Plantar keratoma (nucleated or non-nucleated) beneath a lessor metatarsal head.
2. Depressed metatarsal head in relation to other metatarsal heads.
3. Axial view X-rays indicate a sublocated metatarsal head.
4. Dorsally subluxed proximal phalanx of the affected ray.
5. Localized inflammation in any stage beneath the affected ray.
6. Pathomechanical foot.
7. Enlarged metatarsal head or condyles (not Freibergs).
8. Capsulitis of affected metatarsal-phalangeal joint.

Preoperative Symptoms

1. Sharp pain on ambulation beneath the affected metatarsal head.

2. Sharp pain upon direct palpation of the lesion.
3. Compensation of affected foot during stance phase of gait.
4. Pain in legs, thigh, or low back from accommodative gait.
5. Tenderness around affected metatarsal-phalangeal joint.

Preoperative X-ray Evaluation

1. No visualization of keratoma on X-ray. (Wire lesions to locate.)
2. Metatarsal head may be enlarged.
3. Excessive metatarsal length.
4. Axial views usually show sublocated metatarsal head in relation to adjacent metatarsal heads.
5. Subluxed metatarsal phalangeal joint may be visualized.
6. Normal metatarsal-phalangeal articulation visualized on dorsal-plantar view.
7. Closure of the epiphysis of the lesser metatarsals should be present.

Biomechanical Evaluation

The contact period in a compensated forefoot varus is generally lengthened by pronation of the subtalar articulation and the midtarsal articulations. Pronation extends this period until the forefoot is able to compensate to reach the supportive surface. Therefore the foot is pronated and mobile at a time when it should be becoming supinated and rigid. In the young with good muscle power the pronation may be overcome, but with fatigue and age the foot is only able to reach a supinated attitude during the swing phase. With pronation of the subtalar articulations and the midtarsal articulations, the 1st ray becomes hypermobile, a shearing force is developed under the 2nd metatarsal head with development of a nucleated plantar keratoma.

Any pathomechanical foot in which there is untimely pronation of the subtalar articulations or midtarsal articulations, 1st or 5th rays, creates excess motion of the metatarsals when they should be fixed rigid lever arms for proper propulsion. The metatarsals have abnormal movement, while the skin is fixed by friction to the weightbearing surface, creating a shearing force in the transverse plane. The shearing force is compounded proportionately to the increase in mobility of the forefoot. Foot types on which plantar keratomas appear include forefoot varus, forefoot valgus, triceps surae equinus, and rearfoot varus.

(The open metaphyseal osteotomy should not be peformed unless the proximal phalanx can be manipulated distally off the metatarsal head and maintained in this position with the foot loaded.)

Surgical Procedure

A linear longitudinal incision approximately 3 cm. in length is made commencing at the metatarsal-phalangeal articulation extending proximally. The incision is deepened and, with medial and lateral reflection of the skin and subcutaneous tissue, the extensor digitorum longus tendon is exposed. An incision commencing at the proximal aspect of the metatarsal-phalangeal joint is made laterally to the extensor tendon, running proximally for 2½ cm. The tendon is underscored minimally and is retracted medially as the skin and subcutaneous tissues are retracted medially and laterally with a small Weitlander retractor. Thus the dorsal aspect of the neck of the metatarsal and the most dorsal proximal aspect of the metatarsal head are exposed. With minimal dissection, the sides of the distal aspect of the metatarsal neck is exposed and the bone is scored. A 2″ x 4″ x 1″ sterile wooden block is then held beneath the plantar forefoot to support the metatarsal parabola during the osteotomy. Using a 16 oz. Rush mallet and a 1 cm. Lombodi osteotome held perpendicular to the long axis of the metatarsal, the shaft is transsected obliquely, 5-10 degrees from the transverse plane, with the medial aspect of the osteotomy being most proximal, through the metaphysis (anatomical neck). This frees the metatarsal head which is not fixed, but allowed to seek its proper level upon ambulation. The plantar aspect of the intact metatarsal shaft is then inspected to be certain there are no protruding plantar osseous structures. If part of the lateral plantar condyle was cut through, it should be removed from the metatarsal shaft and rasped smooth. The retractor is then released and the vital structures are realigned. The extensor tendon is then identified and may be lengthened using a "Z" tendon slide if desired. The surgical site may then be closed with 2 3-0 Dexon subcutaneous sutures. The skin is opposed and maintained with several simple 5-0 nylon sutures. ½ cc. of Decadron is then injected into the osteotomy site following closure. One 4 x 4 gauze sponge is folded in half and placed longitudinally beneath the head and shaft of the 5th metatarsal. Adaptic is placed over the surgical site and three 4 x 4 gauze sponges placed over the surgical site and maintained in position with 2″ sterile Kling. If the procedure is performed in the hospital, ambulation is allowed in a surgical shoe the following day. When the surgery is performed in the office, the patient must ambulate immediately with the surgerized foot in a surgical shoe.

Postoperative Management

1. Sterile compression dressing.
2. 24 hour ambulation to allow head to seek its proper level dorsally.

3. Reece shoe for 2-3 weeks following surgery to affected foot.
4. Analgesic of choice.
5. Postoperative X-rays at 10 days to assure alignment.
6. Weekly visits to office following surgery for 5 weeks, then once a month for 2 months.
7. Suture removal at 14-21 days.
8. Follow with biomechanical exam and fabrication of orthotics.

Advantages

1. Visualization of bone to be surgerized.
2. Maintenance of length pattern of metatarsal parabola.
3. Maintenance of proper spacing between metatarsal heads, as opposed to a metatarsal head resection.
4. Technique is simpler than most other metatarsal osteotomies.
5. No casting necessary.
6. Patient may ambulate immediately after surgery in surgical shoe.
7. Painful intractible plantar keratomas will disappear within 3 to 12 weeks following surgery.
8. Technique is easily performed in office.
9. Minimal swelling and bone callous with steroid injected into osteotomy site. Some patients require no analgesic following steroid injection into surgical site.

Disadvantages

1. Abnormal displacement of head may occur with short immobilization.
2. Pseudoarthrosis.
3. Rotation of head may cause pain.
4. Infection.
5. Excessive dorsal swelling.
6. Allergic reaction to suture material.
7. Non-union or delayed union from improper or abbreviated immobilization in surgical shoes.
8. Not to be performed on subluxed metatarsal-phalangeal joints. Where the subluxation will restrict the dorsal movement of the metatarsal other techniques should be considered.
9. No change in position of metatarsal head.
   COMMENT: It cannot be over emphasized that the patient must walk on the surgerized foot (feet) to allow the retrograde forces of the weight bearing surface to move the freed metatarsal head dorsally.
10. Transfer lesions.

A-C show an open metaphyseal osteotomy of the 5th metatarsal using the Lombodi osteotome and mallet. Note that the site of the osteotomy transection is on an angle at the surgical neck of the metatarsal with the cut more distal laterally. This enables the head of the metatarsal to slide medially as well as dorsally. This also repairs a mild Tailor's bunion.

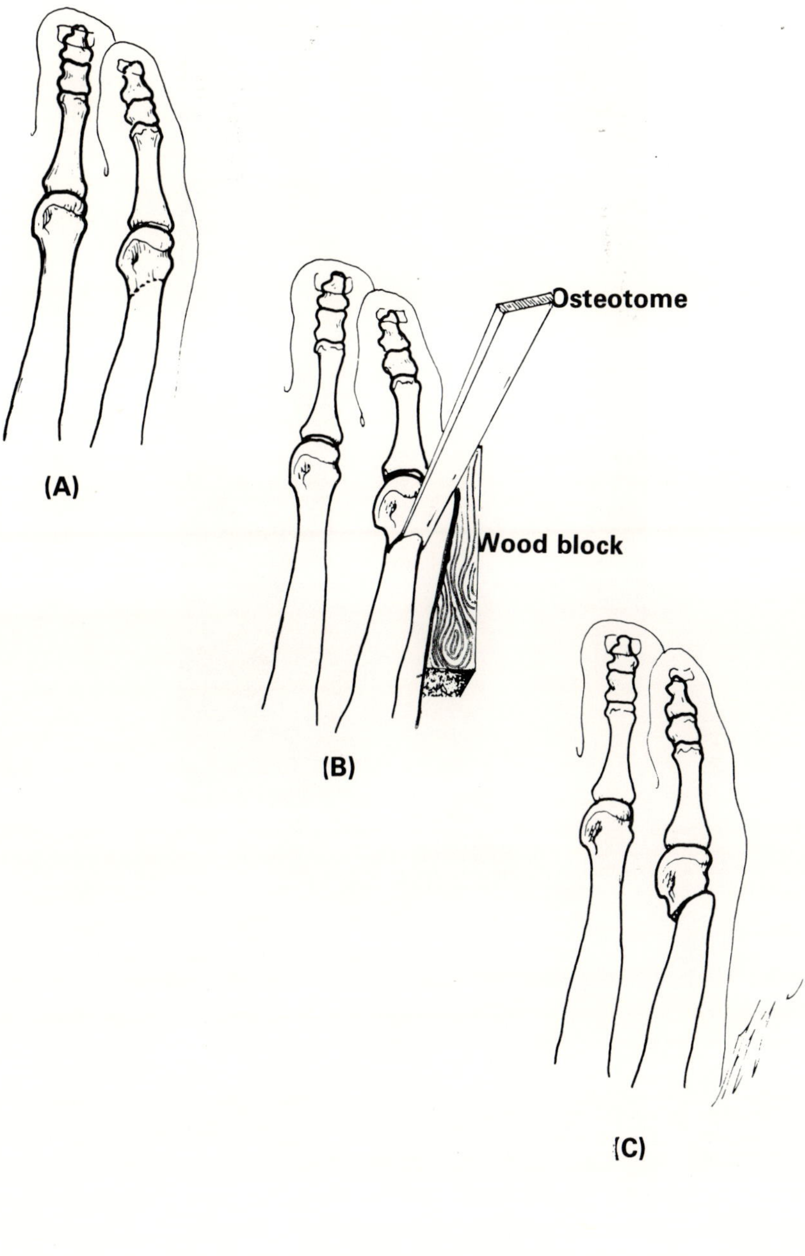

FIGURE 1
OSTEOCLASIS-TYPE PROCEDURE

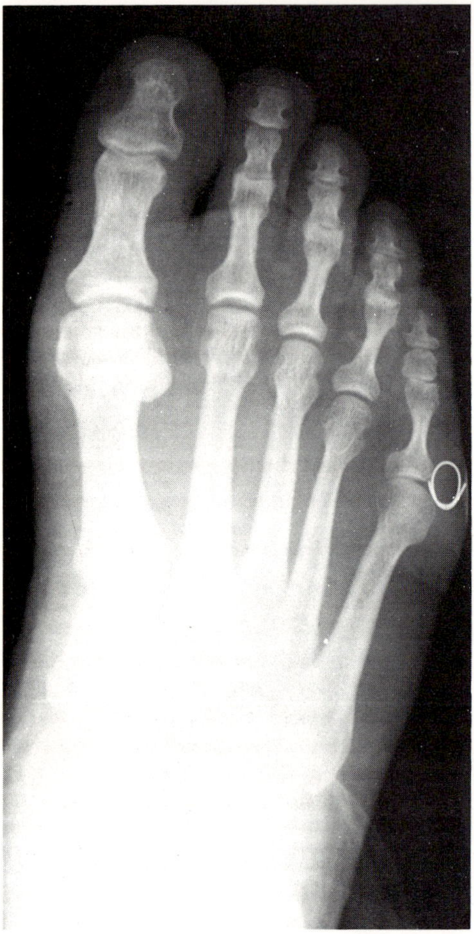

FIGURE 2A
PREOPERATIVE X-RAY

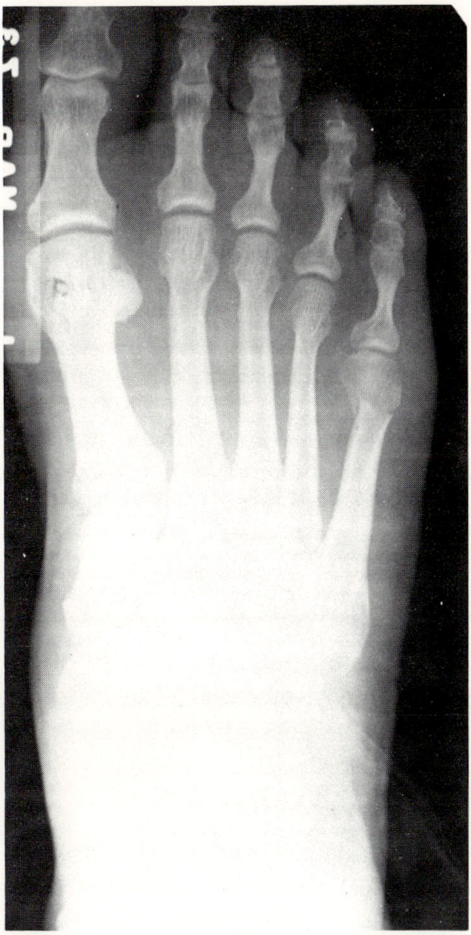

FIGURE 2B
POSTOPERATIVE X-RAY

5. Plantar Condylectomy

Plantar condylectomy for a sub fifth metatarsal lesion is not commonly employed in podiatric surgery. The procedure employs the resection of the plantar portion of the metatarsal head.

Preoperative Signs

1. An intractable plantar tyloma on the plantar aspect of the fifth metatarsal head.
2. A plantarly positioned fifth metatarsal.
3. An apparent shortened fifth ray.

Preoperative Symptoms

1. Painful plantar callous sub fifth metatarsal head.
2. Inability to wear proper footgear comfortably.
3. No pain on range of motion of the fifth metatarsal-phalangeal joint.

Biomechanical Evaluation

1. Forefoot varus or supinatus is usually present.
2. The fifth ray range of motion dorsally is still below four.
3. The fifth toe may be dorsally contracted.

Preoperative X-ray Evaluation

1. Possible signs of forefoot varus are present.
2. There should be evidence of a deformed enlarged plantar condyle.
3. No degenerative joint disease present.

Surgical Procedure

The approach used for a plantar condylectomy of the fifth metatarsal differs from that described for a head resection or a lateral condylectomy. Since the plantar aspect of the metatarsal head must be visualized in this procedure, the approach must be more lateral. There are more tendinous and muscular structures encountered beneath the subcutanous tissue. An incision is made extending from mid-shaft of the proximal phalanx to mid-shaft of the fifth metatarsal. The Abductor digiti quinti must be reflected from the capsular area, and a linear lateral capsulotomy is performed. The soft tissue structures are dissected from the head, exposing the plantar condyle. Removal of the plantar condyles may be accomplished with an osteotome and mallet, or a rotary bone saw. The condyles should be removed flush with the shaft of the metatarsal plantarly. All sharp projections are rasped smooth, and the area flushed with sterile solution (Fig. 1).

Capsular closure is accomplished with chromic or Dexon suture. Skin closure is always made with either single interrupted sutures or vertical mattress sutures, since there is a great deal of stress on the incision line postoperatively.

Postoperative Management

The patient is allowed to ambulate as soon as possible in a postoperative shoe. Suture removal is accomplished in approximately two weeks or longer, depending on the stress of the incision. The patient may return to shoes in two to 4 weeks.

Advantage

1. Preserves the length of the ray.

Disadvantages

1. Lesion recurrence
2. Postoperative arthritis
3. Postoperative fracture of the metatarsal shaft

This shows the portion of bone to be removed in the performance of a plantar condylectomy.

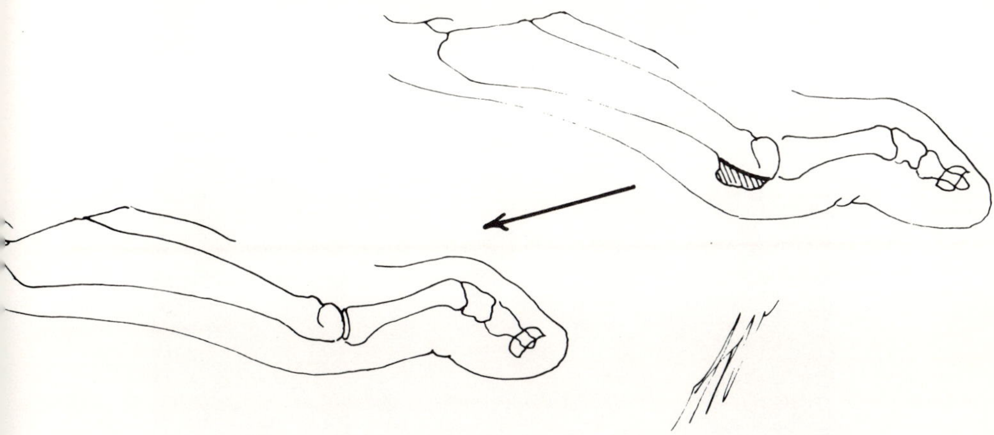

FIGURE 1
PLANTAR CONDYLECTOMY

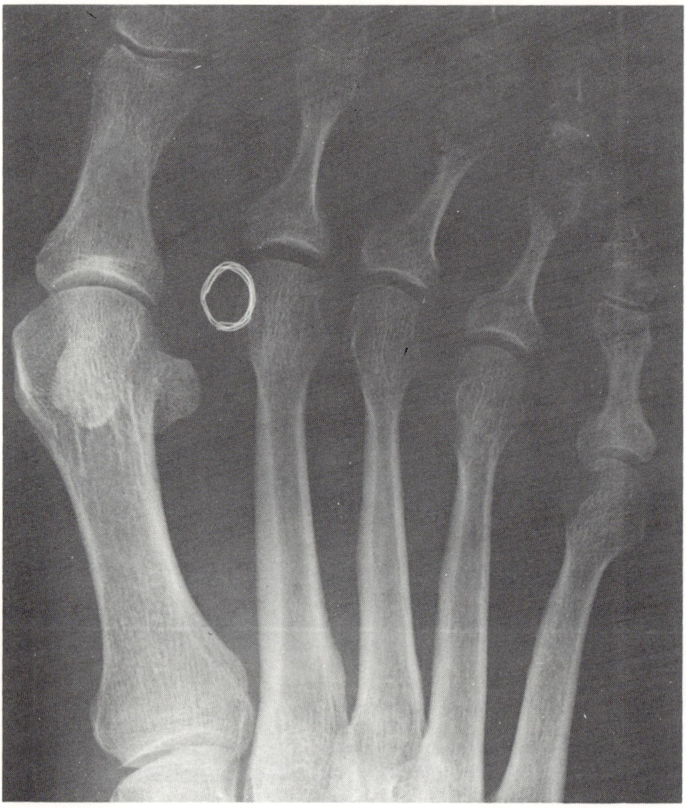

FIGURE 2A
PREOPERATIVE DORSO PLANTAR X-RAY
Note the enlarged plantar condyle of the second metatarsal.

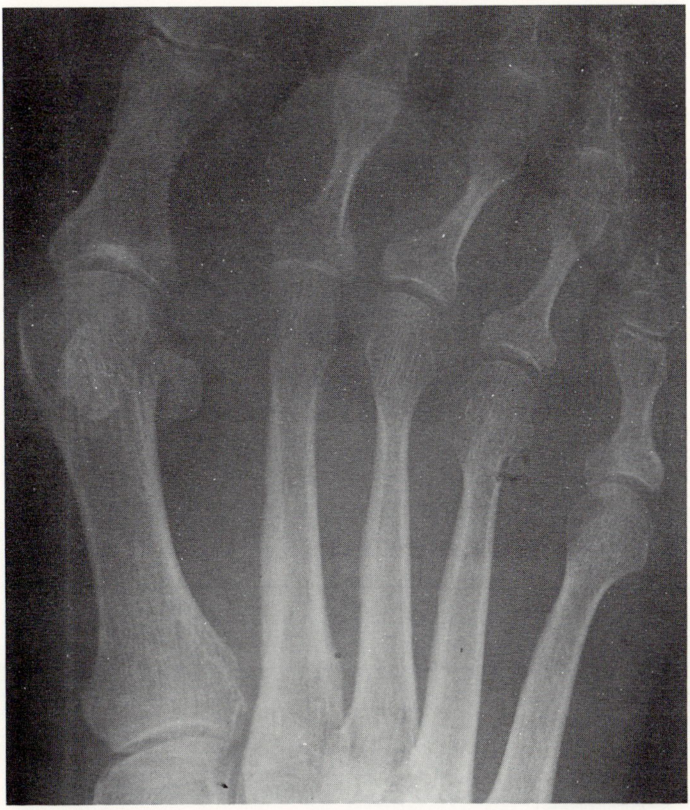

FIGURE 2B
POSTOPERATIVE DORSO PLANTAR X-RAY
Note the postoperative appearance of the plantar condylectomy.

6. Lateral Condylectomy

Occasionally, deformities of the fifth metatarsal are not always just positional in nature. There are occasions that present an enlargement in the structure of the bone. When this is coupled with an abnormal position, it is sometimes necessary to consider removal of the offending enlargement of bone as the procedure of choice. Such is the case with the lateral condylectomy. This procedure should be considered when there is obvious enlargement of the lateral condyle, or a "Tailor's Bunion" present, and the surgeon wishes to preserve the weight bearing function of the fifth metatarsal.

Preoperative Signs

1. A lateral tyloma with or without an underlying bursa.
2. No plantar projection or prominence of the metatarsal.
3. A fifth toe varus position or a "Tailor's bunion."
4. A laterally prominent fifth metatarsal head.

Preoperative Symptoms

1. Pain at the fifth metatarsal head laterally.
2. Pain is elicited on lateral pressure, and is accentuated in footgear.
3. No pain on range of motion of the fifth toe.

Biomechanical Evaluation

1. Minimal forefoot varus present.
2. Hypermobile fifth ray in gait.
3. A pronated foot in gait; usually no equinus.
4. A dorsiflexed and abducted fifth metatarsal, with an associated adducted fifth toe.

Preoperative X-ray Evaluation

1. X-ray signs of a pronated foot at the mid-tarsal joint.
2. Enlarged or prominent lateral condyle of the fifth metatarsal head.
3. No degenerative joint disease present.
4. A congruous joint with an associated fifth toe varus.

Surgical Procedure

This procedure employs the removal of a portion of the fifth metatarsal head in an effort to correct a structural defect at the fifth metatarsal-phalangeal joint. As such, the primary aim of surgery is to remove the abnormal bone without destroying the integrity of the joint. In this procedure, it is essential that the articular cartilage that is effective be preserved for function. The approach is made in a dorso-lateral fashion so as to encounter as few structures as possible. The subcutaneous tissue is dissected revealing the tendinous insertion of the extensor digitorum longus. The length of the incision extends from the base of the proximal phalanx to the upper one third of the shaft of the metatarsal. The capsular incision will vary with the deformity present. If it is primarily an enlarged condyle, a linear capsulotomy is performed, if it is a "Tailor's bunion" then a "U" shaped capsulotomy may be performed in an effort to correct the varus toe.

Removal of the offending condyle is usually performed with an osteotome or rotary bone saw from distal to proximal with the cut flush with the shaft. The remaining sharp dorsal and plantar edges may be rasped smooth, and flushed with sterile solution.

Capsular closure is affected with single interrupted chromic or Dexon sutures whether the incision is linear of "U" shaped. Skin closure is accomplished with 4-0 or 5-0 nylon sutures.

Postoperative Management

The patient is placed either in postoperative shoes, or in a cut-out shoe for a period of 2-4 weeks. Suture removal is accomplished in fourteen days.

Advantages

1. Preservation of the joint function.
2. Removal of the pathologic portion of bone.
3. Relief of symptoms, and correction of a varus fifth toe.

Disadvantages

1. Possible postoperative arthritis.
2. Recurrence of deformity if foot control is not established.
3. Should not be performed in the presence of an intact epiphysis.

This shows the portion of bone to be removed in the performance of a lateral condylectomy.

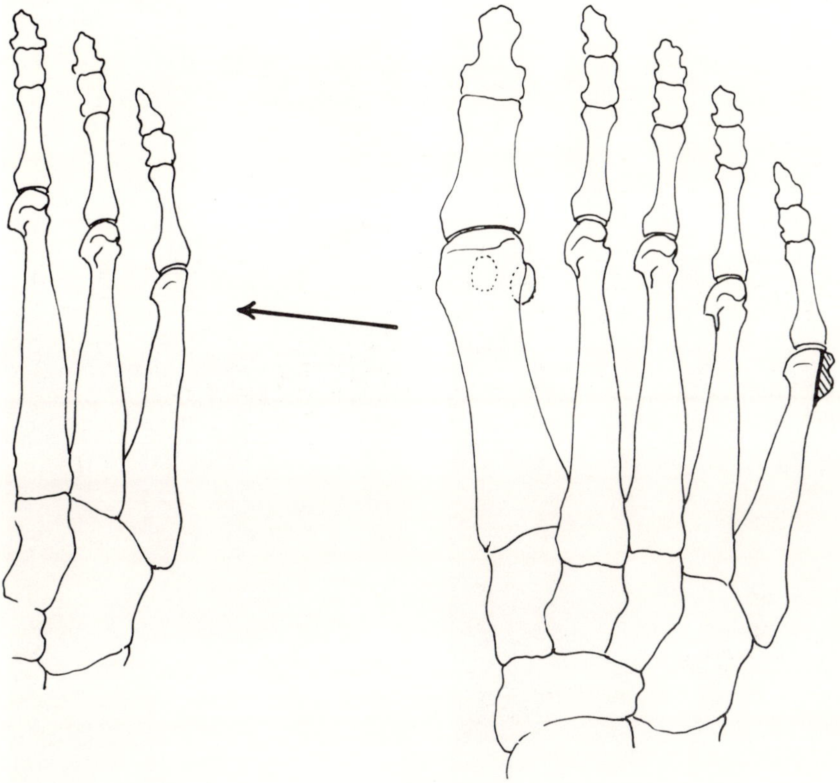

FIGURE 1
LATERAL CONDYLECTOMY

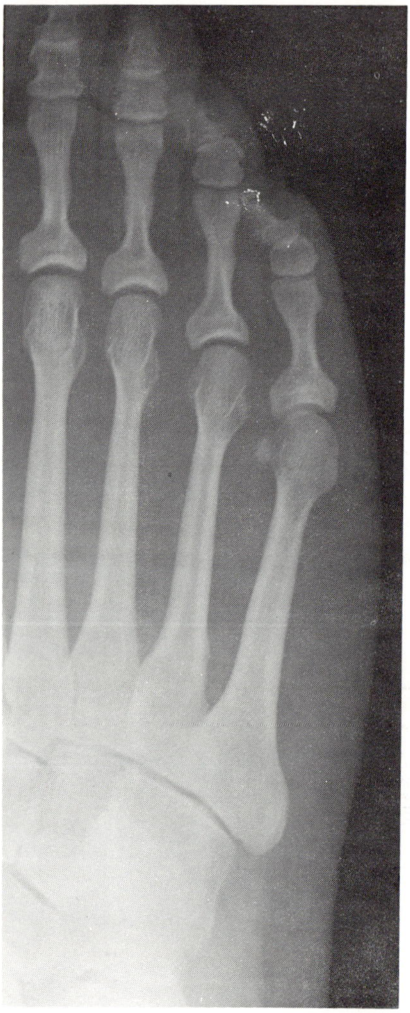

FIGURE 2A
PREOPERATIVE X-RAY

Note the enlarge 5th lateral condyle.

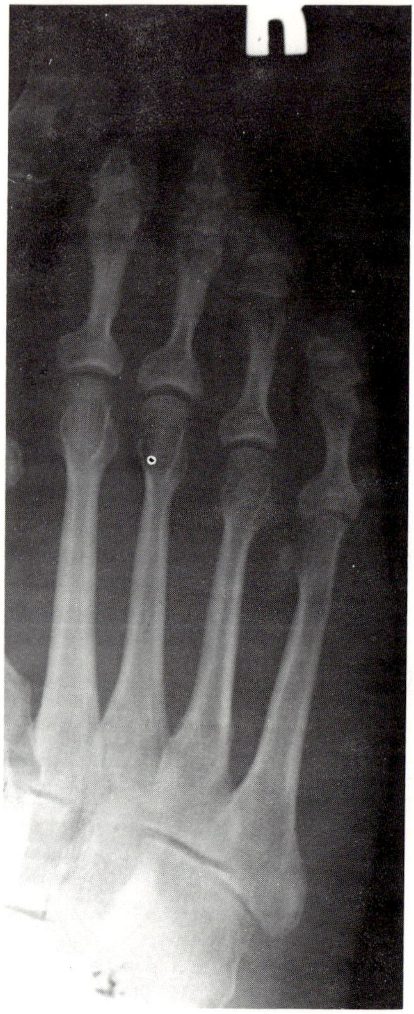

FIGURE 2B
POSTOPERATIVE X-RAY

This X-ray shows the removal of the lateral condyle of the 5th metatarsal.

7. Fifth Metatarsal Head Resection

This procedure deals with the complete removal of the fifth metatarsal head at the surgical neck. The object of the procedure is to remove the entire weight-bearing structure of the fifth metatarsal.

Preoperative Signs

1. An intractable nucleated plantar keratoma on the plantar aspect of the fifth metatarsal.
2. A shearing keratoma on the lateral aspect of the fifth metatarsal.
3. A deviated fifth metatarsal-phalangeal joint or "Tailor's Bunion".
4. Inflamed bursa at the lateral margin of the fifth metatarsal head. This may not be present in a chronic condition.
5. Painful range of motion of the fifth metatarsal-phalangeal joint.

Preoperative Symptoms

1. Plantar pain in the area of the fifth metatarsal head.
2. Lateral pain in the area of the fifth metatarsal head.
3. Painful range of motion at the fifth metatarsal-phalangeal joint.
4. Inability to comfortably wear certain types of footgear.
5. Occasionally a positive history of arthritis.

Biomechanical Evaluation

1. Rearfoot varus may or may not be present.
2. Forefoot varus or a supinatus due to equinus is almost always present.
3. The fifth ray range of motion dorsally is still below the level of four.
4. The fifth digit is in a varus position.

Preoperative X-ray Evaluation

1. Irregularity in the size or shape of the fifth metatarsal head is seen.
2. Fifth toe varus or Tailor's bunion is seen occasionally.
3. The signs of a forefoot varus or supinatus are present.
4. Arthritic signs may be present.

Surgical Procedure

Resection of the fifth metatarsal head is a relatively common procedure in forefoot surgery. The procedure as described has two main points of concern surgically. They are the location of the incision, and the angle at which the metatarsal head is removed.

The skin incision is placed at the dorso-lateral aspect of the fifth metatarsal-phalangeal joint, extending in a curvo-linear fashion from mid-shaft of the proximal phalanx to mid-shaft of the fifth metatarsal.

The subcutaneous tissue is dissected revealing the expansion of the extensor tendon at the fifth metatarsal-phalangeal joint. It is not generally necessary to selectively lengthen this tendon since you are in effect shortening the ray.

The capsule of the fifth metatarsal-phalangeal joint is in the same plane as the tendon and it is incised longitudinally. The ligamentous structures between the head and the base are excised, exposing the entire fifth head.

The fifth metatarsal is now cut at the surgical neck at the following angles. First, the cut is made so as to remove more lateral bone than medial, and then more plantar bone than dorsal. The method used to resect the head is not vital, and therefore is left to the surgeons discretion. Usually, osteotomes or power equipment is used since this leaves the cleanest cut. The metatarsal head is then sharply dissected free.

All edges are rasped smooth and flushed with a sterile solution so that the remaining portion of the metatarsal is free of any sharp edges. The capsule is closed with chromic or Dexon sutures usually employing an hour glass type closure. The subcutaneous tissue is closed in layers being careful to ligate all obvious severed vessels. Skin closure is then accomplished.

Postoperative Management

The patient is placed in a postoperative shoe, and early ambulation is encouraged. Ace bandages may be used in an effort to contain the postoperative edema. Suture removal follows in two weeks with the patient returning to regular footgear in 2-4 weeks.

Advantages

1. Removal of an abnormal weight bearing structure.
2. Corrects both plantar and lateral lesions.
3. May be performed with a minimal amount of trauma.
4. Allows a varus forefoot to be placed in posted orthotics.
5. Effectively eliminates a painful joint surface.

Disadvantages

1. Must not be performed in young patients with intact epiphysis.
2. May get retraction of the fifth toe.
3. Should not usually be considered in presence of a short fifth toe.
4. Joint destruction.

Shows the approximate angle from lateral to medial of the resection of the metatarsal head.

Shows the surfaces of bone rasped smooth prior to capsular closure.

Shows the relative increase in tendon length after a Metatarsal Head Resection.

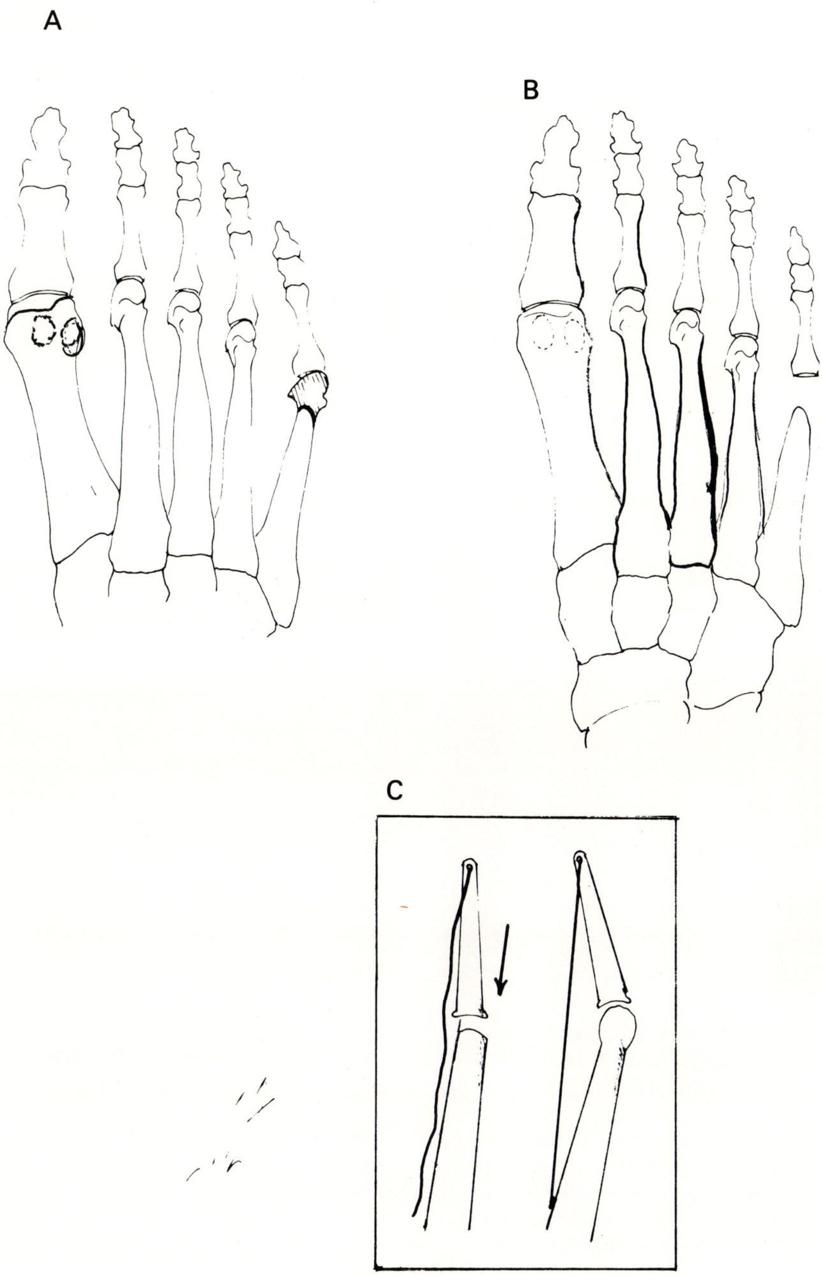

FIGURE 1
FIFTH METATARSAL HEAD RESECTION

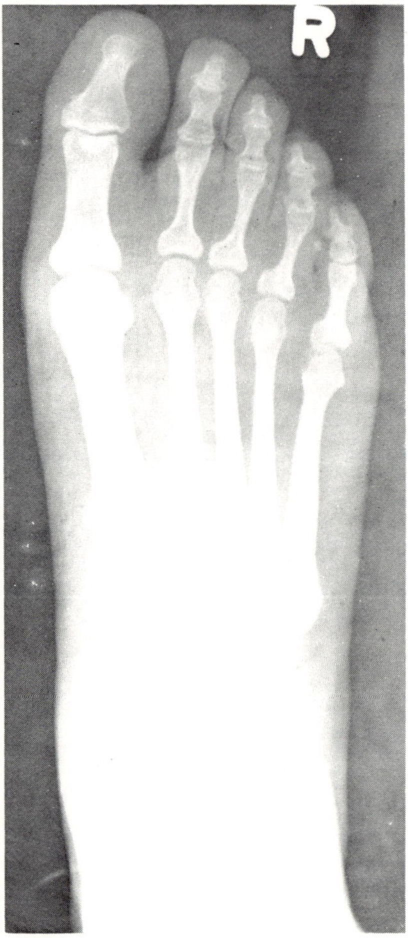

FIGURE 2A
PREOPERATIVE DORSO
PLANTAR X-RAY

This is a preoperative dorso plantar view of a fifth metatarsal head resection. This X-ray shows lateral bowing of the shaft of the metatarsal consistent with a hypermobile fifth ray.

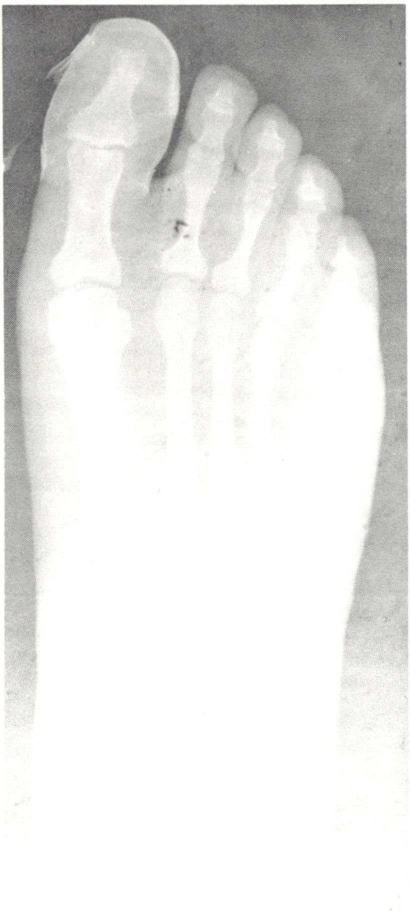

FIGURE 2B
POSTOPERATIVE X-RAY
PLANTAR X-RAY

This is a postoperative view of a fifth metatarsal head resection performed at the neck of the bone.

Bibliography

Davies, H.: Metatarus quintus valgus. *Br. Med. J.,* **1**:664, 1949.

Gerbert, J., Sgarlato, T. E. and Subotnick, S. I.: Preliminary study of a closing wedge osteotomy of the fifth metatarsal for correction of a Tailor's Bunion deformity. *J.A.P.A.* **62**:212-218, 1972.

Hicks, J. H.: Mechanics of the foot. I. The joints. *J. Anat.,* **87**:345, 1953.

McKeever, D. C.: Excision of the fifth metatarsal head. *Clin. Orthop.,* **13**:321, 1959.

Brown, J. E.: Functional and cosmetic correction of metatarsus latus (splayfoot). *Clin. Orthop.,* **14**:166, 1959.

Kelikian, H.: *Hallux Valgus, Allied Deformities of the Forefoot and Metatarsalgia.* W. B. Saunders, Philadelphia, 1965, p. 327.

DuVries, H. L.: *Surgery of the Foot.* The C. V. Mosby Company, St. Louis, 1973.

Amberry, T. R.: *Principles and Practice of Podiatry.* Edited by F. Weinstein, Lea & Febiger, Philadelphia, 1968, p. 167.

McGlamry, D. E.: *A Monograph on Foot Surgery.* Peachtree Podiatry Group, Atlanta, 1969, p. 18.

Sgarlato, T. E.: *Compendium of Podiatric Biomechanics.* California College of Podiatric Medicine, San Francisco, 1971, p. 381.

D. Pan Metatarsal Head Resection for IPK

Resection of all metatarsal heads can be a gratifying procedure, both for the doctor and the patient, in certain situations; however it is a procedure which must be performed only when the proper criteria are met. If at all possible only one foot is operated on at a time in order to help reduce the postoperative disability period. At the end of this section various clinical and radiological evidence will be discussed with regard to whether syndactylism of the toes and/or resection of all or part of the proximal phalanges are necessary.

Preoperative Signs

1. Intractable plantar hyperkeratotic lesions located under most of the metatarsal heads.
2. Atrophy of the plantar fat pad beneath the metatarsal heads.
3. Ability to palpate prominent metatarsal heads.
4. Dorsally contracted toes at the metatarsal-phalangeal joints.
5. Possible contracted toes and proximal interphalangeal joint or distal interphalangeal joint with associated lesions.
6. Range of motion at the metatarsal-phalangeal joint may be limited and painful or may be absent.
7. Range of motion of the metatarsal-phalangeal joint may elicit crepitation.
8. Patient ambulates with an apropulsive type gait.
9. Signs of degenerative disease and deformity in other joints of the body.
10. Ulceration, sub-metatarsal head area.

Preoperative Symptoms

1. Moderate to severe pain on the plantar aspect of the forefoot when the patient ambulates with or without shoe gear.
2. Painful multiple hyperkeratotic lesions on the plantar aspect of the forefoot.

3. Patient may complain of plantar ulcer or ulcers under the metatarsal head areas.
4. Patient may complain of painful dorsally contracted toes when wearing foot gear.
5. Patient complains of pain when most of the metatarsal-phalangeal joints are moved.
6. Patient may complain that the toes can not be moved or straightened.
7. History of metabolic disease such as rheumatoid arthritis, psoriatic arthritis, etc. is usually given.

Preoperative X-ray Evaluation

1. Evidence of degenerative disease is present.
2. Dorsally contracted metatarsal-phalangeal joint is usually evident.
3. Most of the metatarsal-phalangeal joints show evidence of degenerative changes.
4. Bone loss may be evident at the metatarsal heads secondary to severe degenerative changes.
5. Proliferative changes at the base of the proximal phalanges and/or metatarsal heads may be present.
6. Loss of normal appearing joint space of the majority of the metatarsal-phalangeal joints.
7. Cystic and/or erosive changes of the metatarsal heads may be evident.
8. Generalized osteoporosis may be present.
9. An axial view of the foot will demonstrate prominent metatarsal heads.
10. Moderate to severe angulation deformity of the toes and metatarsal may be present.

Biomechanical Evaluation

1. Patient ambulates with an apropulsive gait.
2. Biomechanically there are no contraindications for this procedure since this procedure destroys the total function of the metatarsal-phalangeal joints.

Surgical Procedure

The following is the procedure for a pan-metatarsal head resection without concomitant digital procedures. Usually three dorsal linear skin incisions are made; however, in certain cases four dorsal linear skin incisions may be necessary for adequate exposure. The first incision is made over the dorsal aspect of the 1st metatarsal-phalangeal joint medial to the extensor hallucis longus tendon. By sharp and blunt dissection the extensor tendon is identified and lengthened. A dorsal linear incision is next made through subcutaneous tissue and capsule. Care is taken to keep all dissection to a minimum. By sharp dissection the tissue is reflected exposing the base of the proximal phalanx and the head of the first metatarsal. In most cases not only is the metatarsal head resected but also the base of the proximal phalanx. The amount of metatarsal head resected is determined on the preoperative AP X-ray of the foot in which the surgeon attempts to remove the metatarsal heads in such a manner as to maintain a normal metatarsal parabola. The longest metatarsal should be the second, followed by the first and third, followed by the fourth and finally the fifth. Furthermore, the first metatarsal head is resected in such a fashion as to remove more bone medially than laterally. The rough bone edges are smoothed and the area flushed with copious amounts of sterile saline. The surgical site is packed with a wet sponge and direction is turned toward the next skin incision. This is made in the second interspace extending from the digital web proximally to approximately midshaft between the 2nd and 3rd metatarsals. Through this incision one can resect the second and third metatarsal heads. The extensor tendons are usually tenotomized. The second metatarsal head is resected perpendicular to the long axis of its shaft. Every attempt is made to angulate the dorsal-plantar cut on all the metatarsal heads in order to take more off plantar than dorsal. The third metatarsal head is resected with just a mild deviation from its long axis with more being removed laterally. Once again the surgical site is packed with a wet sponge. The final incision is made from the digital web of the fourth interspace extending proximally to approximately midshaft between the 4th and 5th metatarsals. Through this incision the 4th and 5th metatarsal are resected and the extensor tendons are usually tenotomized. The 4th metatarsal head is resected with more being removed laterally than medially and the same with the fifth metatarsal. It's important to ligate or cauterize all major bleeding vessels since one of the major complications of this procedure is the development of hematomas in the dead spaces with resultant painful fibromata. If you can not adequately obliterate all dead spaces then you should pack any large voids for two reasons; to prevent a hematoma from developing and to act as an internal compression to stop the capillary oozing. The subcutaneous tissues are approximated to obliterate all dead spaces using an absorbable suture material. If packing was utilized then one must take care not to suture the packing to soft tissue when closing the subcutaneous tissues. The skin is approximated using 4-0 or 5-0 nylon sutures. A few drops of dexamethasone, is applied to each of the denuded metatarsals which has been found to help minimize the postoperative pain; the foot is then dressed with a sterile compression dressing.

Postoperative Management

The patient is kept at complete bed rest for at least 24 to 36 hours. If a compression bandage was utilized it is released 24 hours postoperatively. The patient can begin ambulating approximately 36 to 48 hours postoperatively wearing an ace bandage on the foot and leg to help minimize the edema and a wooden surgical shoe. If packing was used at the time of surgery then it is usually removed approximately two to three days postoperatively under sterile conditions. Sutures are removed in 14 to 21 days postoperatively and the patient can usually return to regular foot gear in approximately 4 weeks postoperatively. The patient should be instructed in ways to help keep the edema in the foot to a minimum for the first two to three weeks postoperatively; i.e. avoiding prolonged dependent positions of the affected leg and foot and the proper application of an ace bandage on the foot and leg.

Advantages

1. Elimination of painful metatarsal-phalangeal joints.
2. Ability of patient to ambulate without the moderate to severe pain that was present preoperatively.
3. Allow patient to wear regular shoe gear.
4. Reduction of dorsally contracted toes in most cases.
5. Elimination of internal pressure to the plantar aspect of the forefoot.

Disadvantages

1. Loss of propulsive gait.
2. Flail toes postoperatively.
3. High incidence of hematoma formation with resulting fibromas.
4. Painful fibrotic areas where the metatarsal head previously existed.
5. Destroys function of metatarso-phalangeal joints.
6. Loss of digital stability.

Considerations for Syndactylism and/or Partial or Complete Proximal Phalangectomy

If one must excise large amounts of the metatarsals and one is already dealing with short toes particularly the fifth, the syndactylism can help reduce further shortening and retraction postoperatively. Also, the syndactylism will aid in achieving some stability of the area distal to the forefoot. Furthermore, if much bone must be removed from the toes a syndactylism may certainly be needed for the above mentioned reasons and to prevent a flail toe which can become a nusiance to the patient postoperatively. With regard to excising all or a portion of the proximal phalanx one must first determine if the phalanx will produce symptoms postoperatively if allowed to remain. Many times the base of the proximal phalanx has undergone proliferative degenerative changes and, without its corresponding metatarsal head present, can easily retract proximally. It thereby becomes the new osseous pressure on the plantar aspect of the forefoot during ambulation. If this is the situation then the offending base should be resected and the toe syndactilized to an adjacent toe.

One also encounters those situations where one or more toes are contracted at the proximal interphalangeal joint with painful keratotic lesions. In these instances it is necessary to perform an arthroplasty at the proximal interphalangeal joint along with the pan metatarsal head resection. Syndactylism is usually not needed unless it was necessary because of above reasons. Finally, one encounters the situation where the proximal phalanx has been so dorsally subluxed at the metatarso-phalangeal joint and ankylosed at the proximal interphalangeal joint that in order to have the toe assume a more natural alignment postoperatively the entire phalanx must be excised. If this must be done then syndactylism to an adjacent toe should be performed.

FIGURE 1

This is a preoperative diagram of the dorsal aspect of the foot showing the placement of the skin incisions. Normally three incisions are used: 1) for resection of the first metatarsal head 2) for resection of the second and third metatarsal heads and 3) for resection of the fourth and fifth metatarsal heads.

FIGURE 2

This diagram shows the *in*correct method for resecting the metatarsal heads. Notice how a normal metatarsal parabola is not created after resection of the metatarsal heads. Also note how each head is resected in the same plane.

FIGURE 3

A. This diagram shows the correct method for resecting the metatarsal heads in order to maintain a normal metatarsal parabola. Also note how the first and fifth metatarsal heads were resected at very oblique angles.

B. Is a lateral view of a metatarsal demonstrating the angulation of metatarsal head resection. Notice how more bone is removed on the plantar surface than on the dorsal surface.

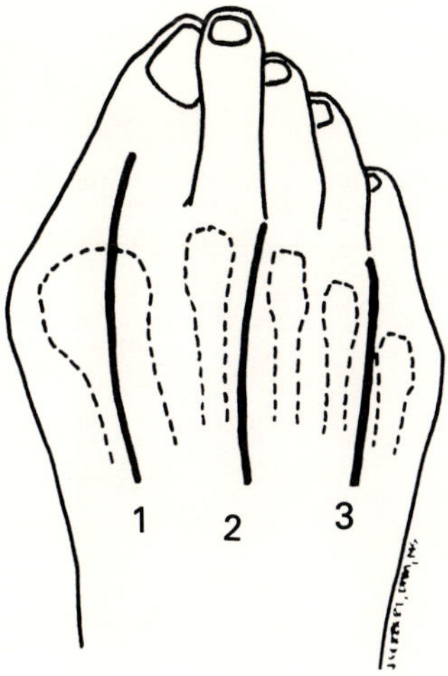

FIGURE 1

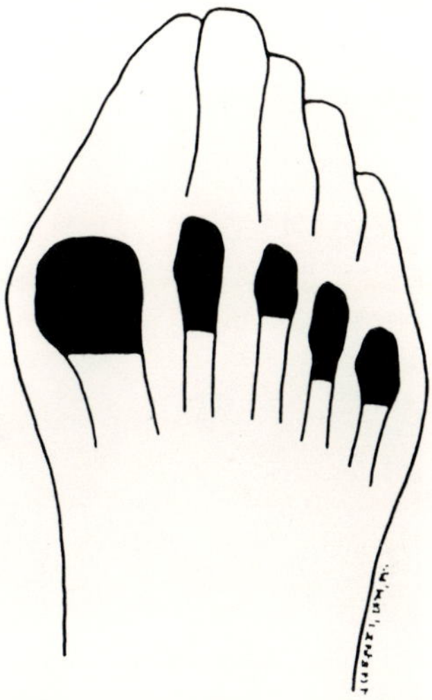

FIGURE 2

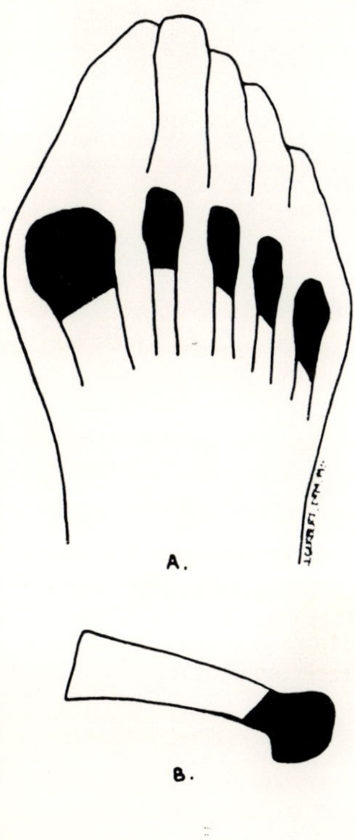

FIGURE 3

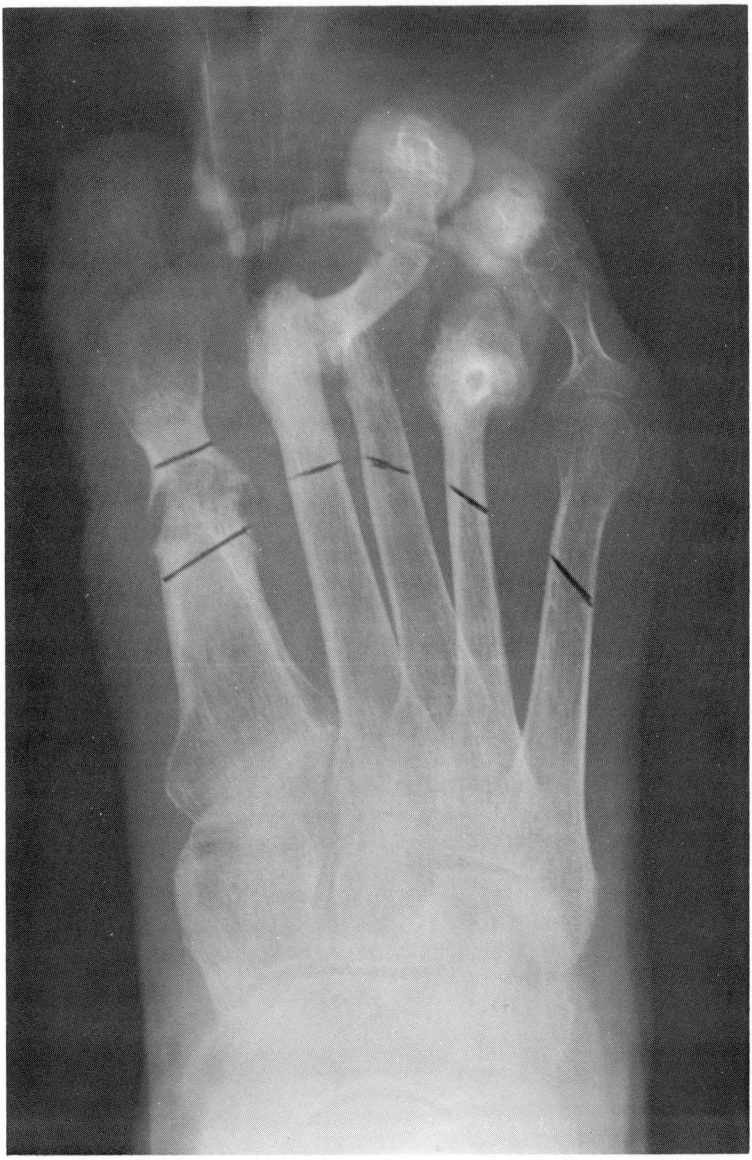

FIGURE 4A
PREOPERATIVE A-P X-RAY

This view demonstrates the severe degenerative changes of the metatarsophalangeal joints secondary to psoriatic arthritis. The only prior surgery on this foot was an amputation of the third toe. Note the severe contractures of the proximal phalanx of the second and fourth toes. The lines drawn on the metatarsals indicate the approximate amount of bone to be resected in order to maintain a parabola.

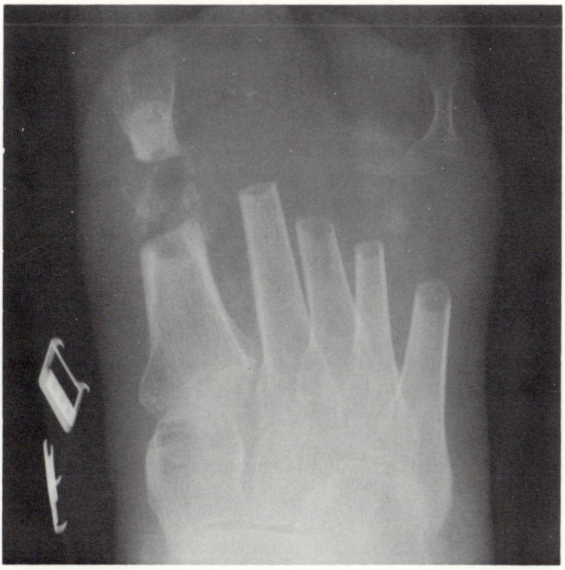

FIGURE 4B
POSTOPERATIVE A-P X-RAY

Following a pan metatarsal head resection. Note that the base of the proximal phalanx of the hallux was resected. The proximal phalanx of the second and fourth toes were excised; the second toe was syndactylized to the hallux and the fourth toe was syndactylized to the fifth toe.

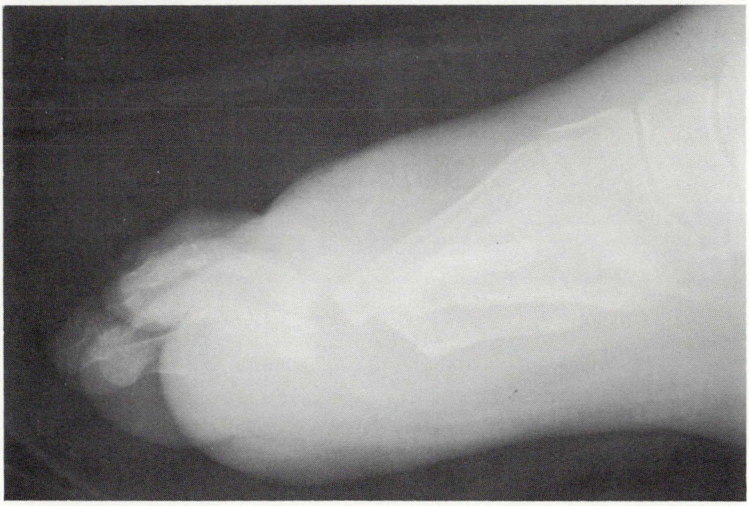

FIGURE 4C
POSTOPERATIVE LATERAL X-RAY

This view demonstrates the angle of the head resection. Note that more bone is removed plantar than dorsal.

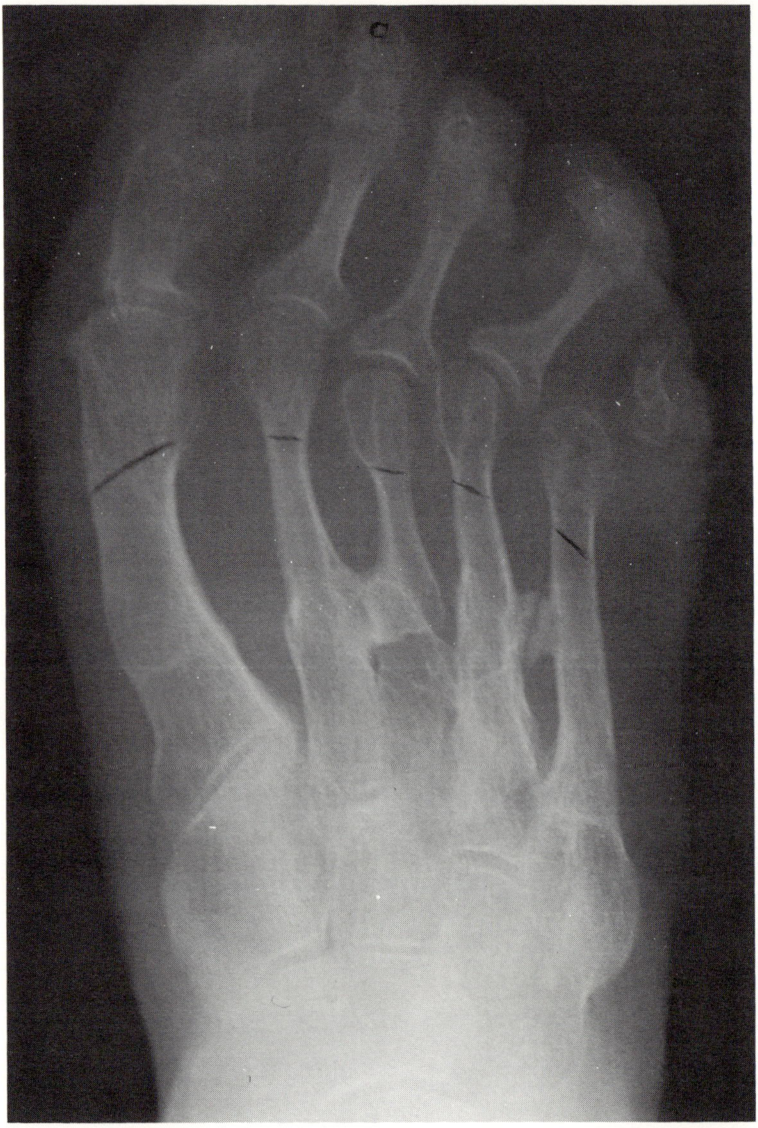

FIGURE 5A
PREOPERATIVE A-P X-RAY

This X-ray demonstrates the degenerative changes of the metatarsophalangeal joints secondary to previous surgical trauma and rheumatoid arthritis. Previous surgery consisted of osteotomy procedures of the metatarsal without fixation, which resulted in exuberant callus formation and bony bridging.

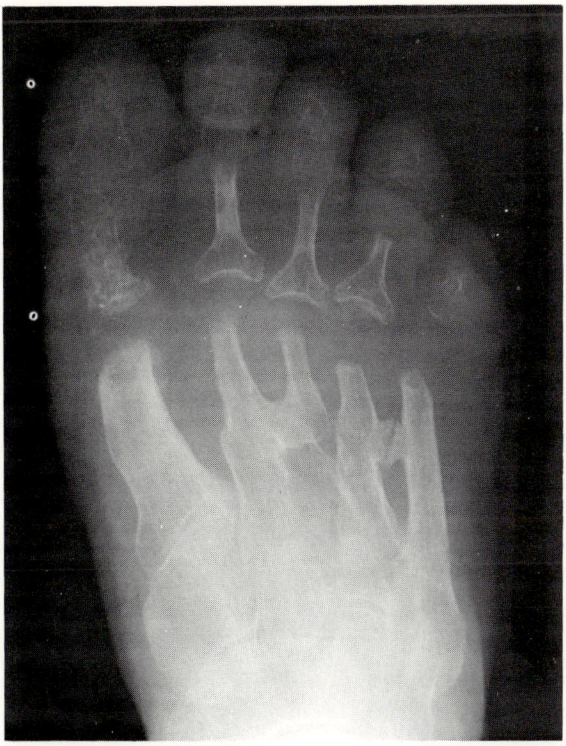

FIGURE 5B
POSTOPERATIVE A-P X-RAY

Following a pan metatarsal head resection and an arthroplasty of the fourth toe. Note how the parabola of the metatarsals was maintained.

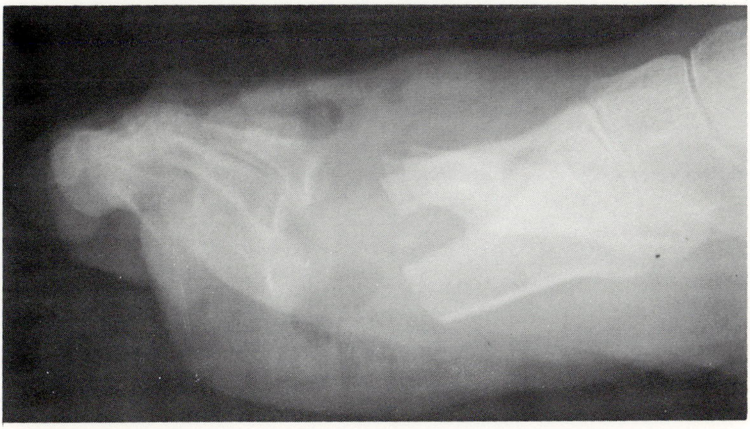

FIGURE 5C
POSTOPERATIVE LATERAL X-RAY

Following a pan metatarsal head resection. Note the angulation of resection of the metatarsal heads with more bone removed plantar than dorsal.

Bibliography

Amuso, S. L., Wissinger, H. A., Margolis, H. M., Eisenbeis, C. H. and Stolzer, B. L.: Metatarsal head resection in the treatment of rheumatoid arthritis, *Clin. Orthop.,* **74**:94-100, 1971.

Barton, N. J.: Arthroplasty of the forefoot in rheumatoid arthritis, *J. Bone Joint Surgery (BR),* **55**:126-33, 1973.

Brattstrom, H. and Brattstrom, M.: Resection of the metatarso-phalangeal joints in rheumatoid arthritis, *Acta. Orthop. Scand.,* **41**:213-24, 1970.

Clayton, M. L.: Surgery of the forefoot in rheumatoid arthritis. *Clin. Orthop.,* **16**:136-140, 1960.

Clayton, M. L.: Surgery of the forefoot in rheumatoid arthritis, *Arthritis & Rheumatism,* **3**:84-85, 1959.

DuVries, Henri L.: *Surgery of the Forefoot,* second edition, C. V. Mosby Co., p. 318-327.

Faithful, D. K. and Savill, D. L.: Review of the results of excision of the metatarsal heads in patients with rheumatoid arthritis, *Ann. Rheum. Dis.,* p. 201-2, 1971.

Giannestras, Nicholas J.: *Foot Disorders–Medical and Surgical Management,* second edition, Lea & Febiger, Philadelphia, 455-464.

Kates, A.: Surgery of the rheumatoid foot, *Proc. Roy. Soc. Med.,* **63**:679-80, 1970.

Kestler, O. C.: Resection of metatarsal heads for metatarsalgia, *Bull. Hosp. Joint Dis.,* **30**:89-100, 1969.

Lipscomb, P. R., Benson, G. M. and Sones, D. A.: Resection of proximal phalanges and metatarsal condyles for deformities of the forefoot due to rheumatoid arthritis, *Clin. Orthop.* **82**:24-31, 1972.

Stess, R. M.: A surgical approach to advanced rheumatoid arthritis of the forefoot, *J.A.P.A.,* **62**:259, 1972.

SECTION IV

SOFT TISSUE PROCEDURES FOR RESOLUTION OF IPK

A. Plantar Excochleation Surgery

This is an ablative technique for the "shelling out" of chronic lesions that have formed in the plantar skin as a consequence of focalized shear and pressure. Excochleation of the intractable plantar keratoma involves blunt surgical extraction of the underlying keratinous plug followed by a marginal saucerization of the wound. Usually performed under local, infiltration anesthesia, this useful ambulatory procedure has been employed by podiatrists for many years.

Though admittedly conservative, this approach to resolution of the intractable plantar keratoma represents a simple clinical solution to the problem. Whereas the focal causative pressure is unaffected by clearance of the secondary lesion, emphasis must be strongly placed on accommodative postoperative control.

Preoperative Signs

The typical isolated keratoma, on the plantar aspect of a metatarso-phalangeal joint, is the general indication for the excochleation procedure.

1. The lesion appears as a heavy, ovoid plantar hyperkeratosis under one of the metatarso-phalangeal joint areas. It is often situated distally over the base of the proximal phalanx.
2. Central metatarsal segments are more commonly affected but, in certain cavus foot types, lesions may develop under the first and fifth segments.
3. On reduction of the overlying hyperkeratomas, a pearly-white disc is revealed below the nucleus; the invaginated top of the "keratinous plug" which is the target of excochleation.
4. Pain can be elicited by direct pressure but the most acute response is obtained by lateral digital compression, as with verrucae.
5. Discriminating manual palpation may reveal a tumorous entity within the plantar tissues. Mobility is restricted by subdermal fixation.

Preoperative Symptoms

The intractable plantar keratoma is discrete and unique as are its symptoms which are far more severe than those of the ordinary plantar metatarsal keratoma. Patients typically describe a gradual progression of pain and disability over a period of several years but some pronounced lesions may develop quite rapidly within months.

1. Pain is experienced only on weightbearing but is largely independent of footgear worn or the type of activity pursued.
2. Lesional reduction only partially relieves the discomfort and disability which rapidly recur due to an accelerated keratogenesis.
3. Patient apprehension, even anxiety, is occasioned by the intense, unpredictable pain produced by stepping upon small irritants.

Biomechanical Evaluation

A comprehensive biomechanical assessment should be performed to reveal underlying musculoskeletal defects suitable for accommodative or reconstructive correction.

Preoperative X-ray Evaluation

As with the need for complete biomechanical study, roentgen appraisal of underlying influences and factors is essential to the preoperative evaluation. Comparative lateral and dorsoplantar weightbearing views, in the individual stance attitude, are taken.

Surgical Procedure

1. The bulk of hyperkeratosis is reduced (Fig. 1).
2. Using the semi-blunt, angled excochleator instrument, insert at the edge of the discernible lesion (Fig. 2).
3. Bluntly circumscribe the periphery of the lesion by a circular, pulling action (Fig. 3).
4. Eventual extirpation and removal of the lesion is accomplished (Fig. 4).
5. The abrupt epidermal margins are then saucerized with the aid of tissue forceps (Fig. 5).
6. Deeper, subcutaneous adhesions, ascertained by skin mobility testing, are divided with the aid of a slender "fibrotome" (Fig. 6).
7. Final appearance of excochleation (Fig. 7).

Postoperative Management

Diligent postoperative attention, to the unaltered causative pressures and biomechanic inducement, is extremely important for a good result. Orthotic control of foot function and metatarsal equilibration should be instituted without delay. Urethane-molded metatarsal sling devices are convenient when dress pumps must be worn. Active digital gripping exercises are prescribed for restoration of digital flexor strength.

Advantages

1. Simple
2. Nondisabling
3. Nondestructive
4. Usually effective when used in combination with functional control and efficient methods of external metatarsal equilibration.

Disadvantages

1. Orthotic control must be maintained.
2. Recurrence of lesion.
3. Does not correct the etiology in most instances.

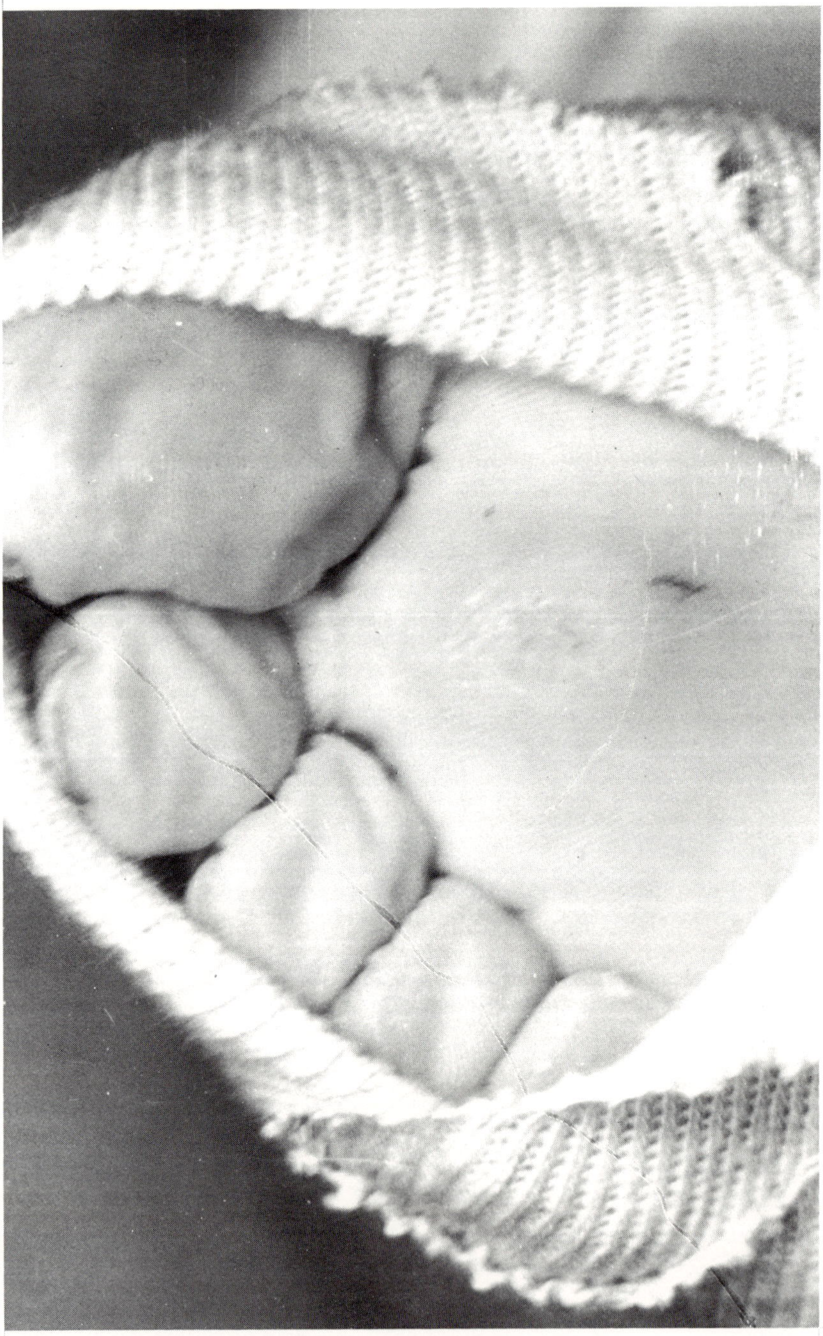

FIGURE 1
Reduction of the bulk of hyperkeratosis

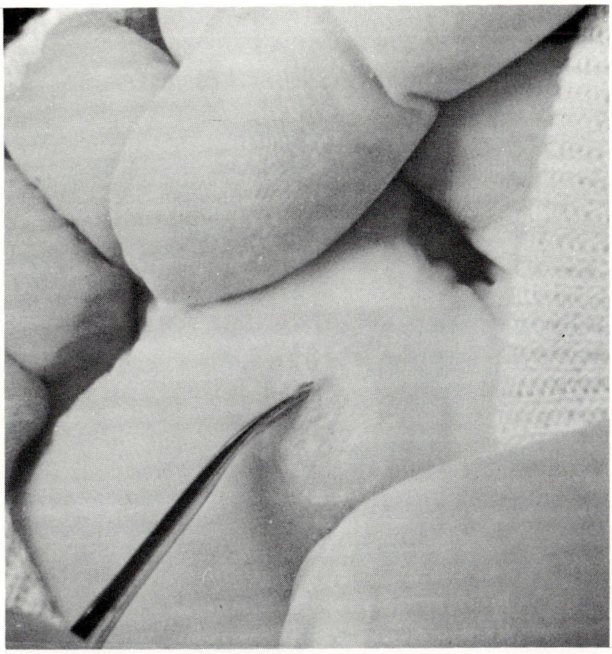

FIGURE 2
Insertion of a semi-blunt, angled excochleator instrument

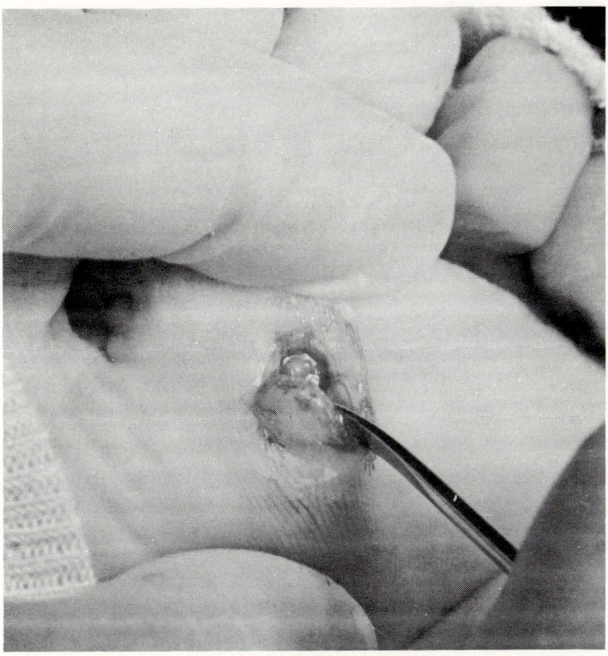

FIGURE 3
Circumscription of the periphery of the lesion

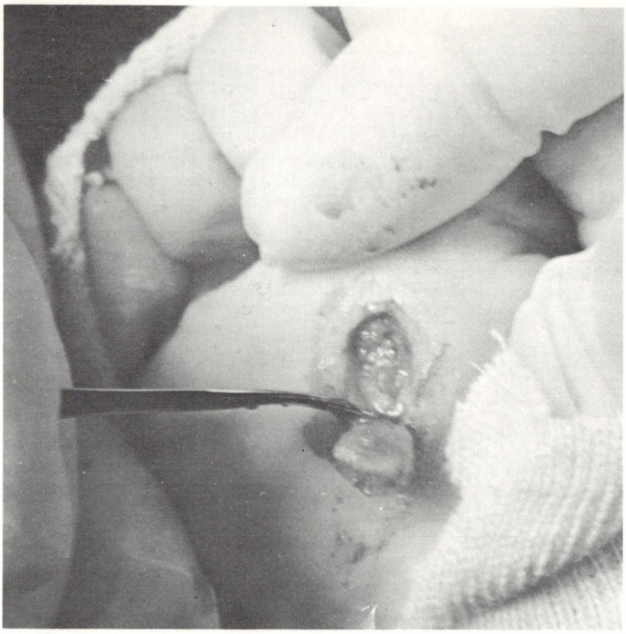

FIGURE 4
Extirpation and removal
of the lesion

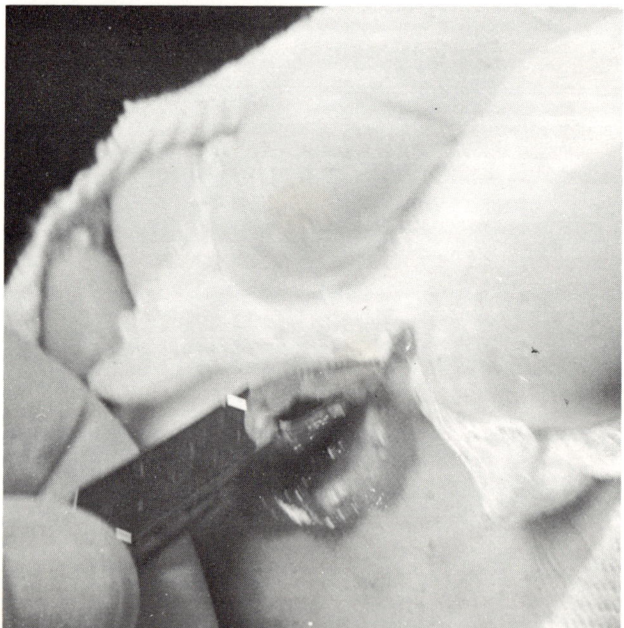

FIGURE 5
Saucerization of the epidermal margins

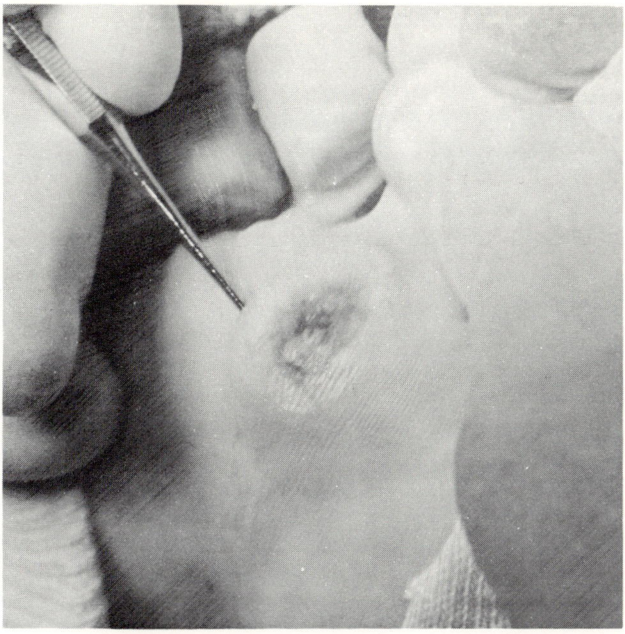

FIGURE 6
Division of deeper, subcutaneous lesions

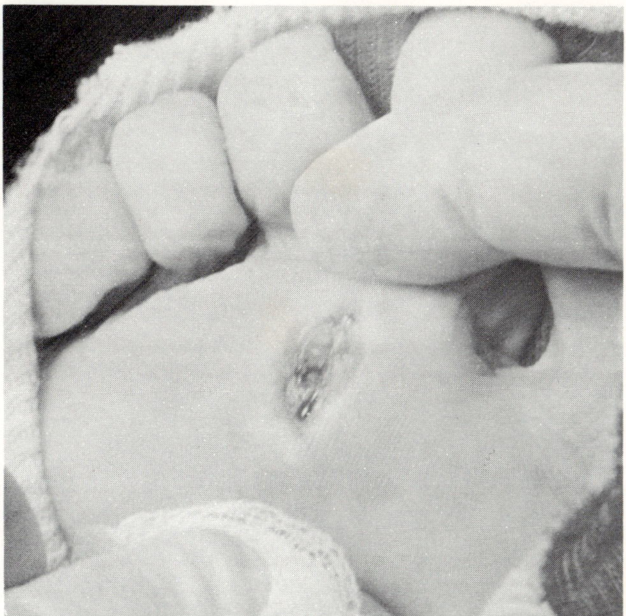

FIGURE 7
Final appearance of excochleation

Bibliography

McGregor, R. R. and Wehr, G. V.: Blunt dissection of plantar verrucae using a new instrument. *J.A.P.A.*, Feb. 1974.

Pringle, W. and Helms, D.: Blunt dissection of verruca plantaris. *Archives of Dermatology,* July, 1973.

Whitney, A. K.: Plantar excochleation technique. *N.E. Journal of Podiatry,* 1973.

Whitney, A. K.: Surgical treatment of the traumatic papilloma. *Current Podiatry,* 1954.

B. Soft Tissue Release Procedures (Tenotomy and Capsulotomy)

These procedures for the reduction of digital tensions and malalignment have been performed as minor operative ventures with varying degrees of success over the years.

General indications for digital release surgery include the mild to moderate static malalignments and tensions secondary to shoe constraint and foot imbalance. Contraindications are the fixed deformities, inherent structural defects, and the inflammatory arthritides. Also less suited are the paralytic, dystrophic, and spastic imbalances affecting the forefoot.

Open or closed approaches to division of tendon and capsular contractures are practiced; the closed release preferable but more difficult to perform. However executed, the simple release of tissue contracture must be persistently maintained to prevent reunion and heightened deformity.

Preoperative Signs

The pendent or dangling foot inevitably exhibits relative dorsiflexion and retraction of the toes which vanishes in the normal stance position. Thus, in the evaluation of digital position and tension one is well advised to place the foot in its simulated stance position at right angles with the leg. Additionally, one should put the foot in strong dorsiflexion, to test for dorsal metatarsophalangeal capsule contractures with the extensor tendons relaxed, and in strong plantarflexed position, to detect any digital flexion contractures with relaxation of the long digital flexor tendons.

Preoperative Tests

1. Pendent (nonweightbearing) Testing
    a. Neutral Position for general appraisal
    b. Forced Dorsiflexion for detection of dorsal metatarsophalangeal contracture
    c. Forced Plantarflexion for detection of plantar interphalangeal contractures
2. Stance (weightbearing) Testing

a. Alignment and taxicity in relaxed, usual attitude of stance
b. Postural centering and test-rebalancing of foot tensions and alignment

Preoperative Symptoms

The symptoms of intractable plantar keratoma, in association with digital tensions and malalignment, stem from secondary forefoot lesions, arthralgia, and functional insufficiency.

1. Associated digital lesions
   a. Dorsal digital lesions with retractive malposition of the toes
   b. Dorsal and distal digital lesions with contraction deformities
2. Metatarso-phalangeal pain
   a. Pain from subluxation and luxation
   b. Limitation of joint motion through marginal distortion and erosion
3. Functional insufficiency related to
   a. Pain-avoidance (lesions)
   b. Tarsal pathomechanics
   c. Leg muscle fatigue and strain

Biomechanical Evaluation

The complete biomechanical appraisal of the feet and lower limbs is essential to an intelligent interpretation of tensions and malalignment of the forefoot. In addition to the aforementioned testing for tendon tensions and capsular contractures, one should carefully consider:

1. Local anatomic defects and abberations by way of segment length, declination, splay, and torsion, and any articular anomalies, alterations, or abnormal set angles. Deviations from normal musculotendinous course or insertion.
2. Footgear influences by way of improper style, fit, flare, shank, or heel height.
3. Tarsal and lower extremity pathomechanical problems affecting forefoot function.
4. Consideration of possible neurotrophic, spastic, paralytic, and myodystrophic disorders.
5. Planning of postoperative orthotics, exercises, and physiatric measures.

Preoperative X-ray Evaluation

The complete, weightbearing X-ray study of the feet, in their individual stance attitude, permits a definitive appraisal of bone-joint configuration and alignment. Specifically, one should observe for any local structural defects or impediments which may obstruct the intended surgical realignment through soft tissue release.

Surgical Procedure

Tendon shortening and capsular contracture can be overcome by "open" or "closed" division. Closed procedure permits only tenotomy and capsulotomy while open approaches facilitate a more versatile repair through tendon tacking, slide-lengthening, and capsulorrhaphy. Because the latter methods are discussed elsewhere in conjunction with open joint reconstruction techniques, we shall deal only with the closed approach in this section.

1. Closed Extensor Release

   Under local infiltration anesthesia, a dorsal stab incision is made with a slender tenotome at the level of, and slightly lateral of, the affected metatarso-phalangeal joint. The tenotome is threaded superficially toward and over the long extensor tendon which is subsequently divided by a firm "sawing motion"(Fig. 2.) During the extensor tendon release,

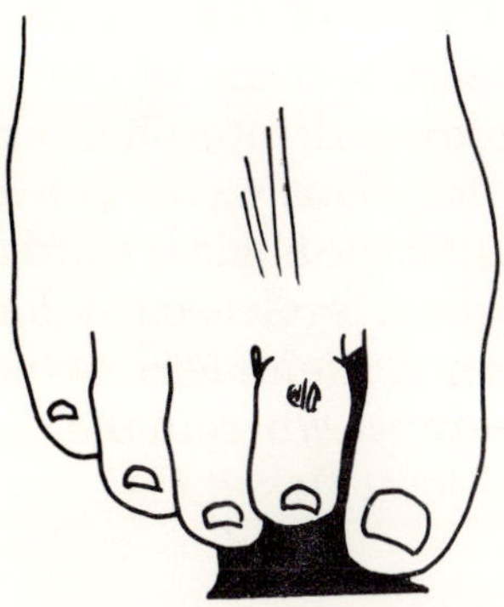

FIGURE 1

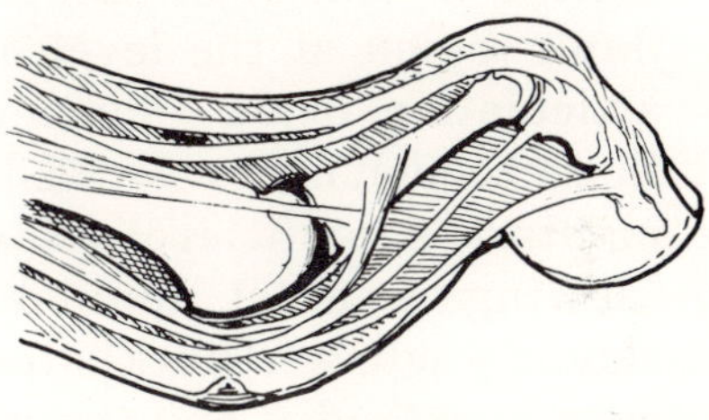

   the tendon is maintained under tension by manual stretching and foot plantarflexion. In most cases, the short extensor tendon must also be divided by a deeper pressure of the tenotome against the dorsolateral aspect of the joint (Fig. 3).

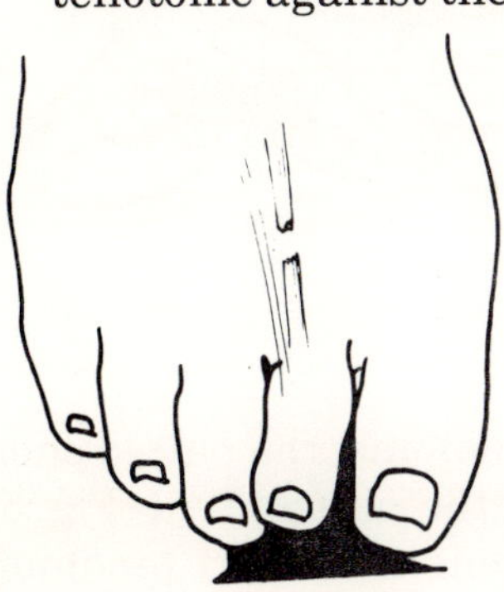

FIGURE 2

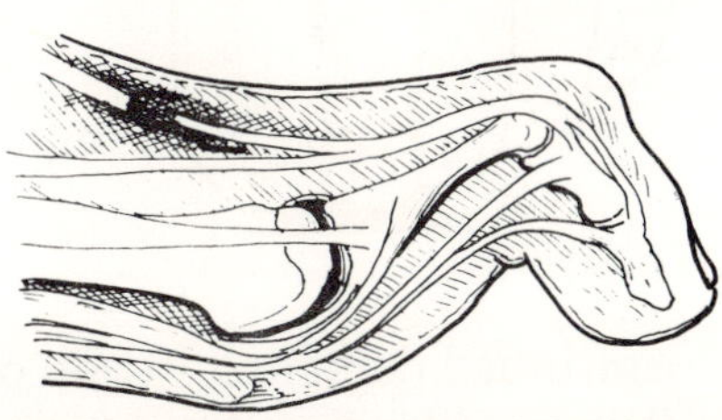

The surgeon then moves the foot into strong dorsiflexion to present the taut dorsal capsules for transection while the digit is firmly plantarflexed to increase capsular resistance (Fig. 3). A good result is gauged by producing a straight toe in the pendent, plantarflexed foot position and a completely plantarflexed digit when the foot is held in its neutral, stance-simulated position.

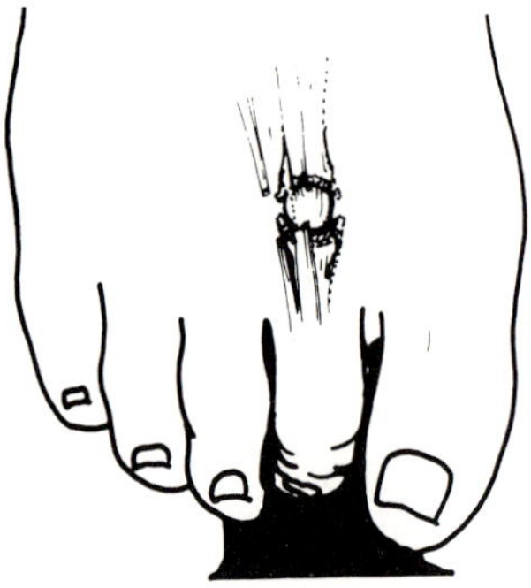

FIGURE 3

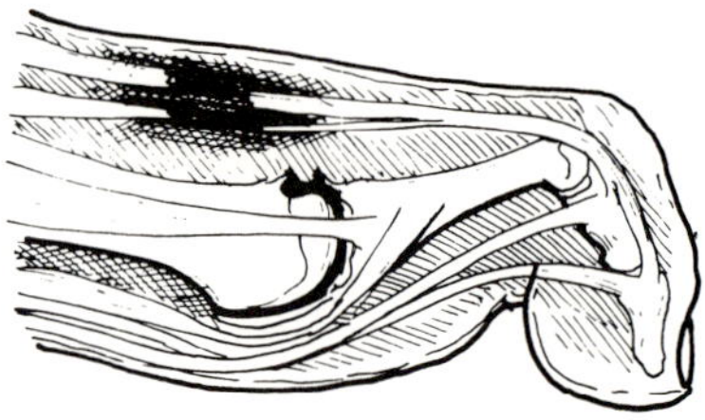

2. Closed Flexor Release
Following local infiltration anesthesia of the contracted digit, a medial or lateral stab incision is made in the mid-flank region at the level of the proximal interphalangeal articulation, using a slender tenotome instrument. The long flexor tendon is first divided by passing the blade toward and plantarly superficial of the tendon which is released by dorsal "sawing" against applied resistance. Complete division should produce a "buckle-toe" appearance wherein the distal joint is extended and the proximal joint flexed (Fig. 4). By

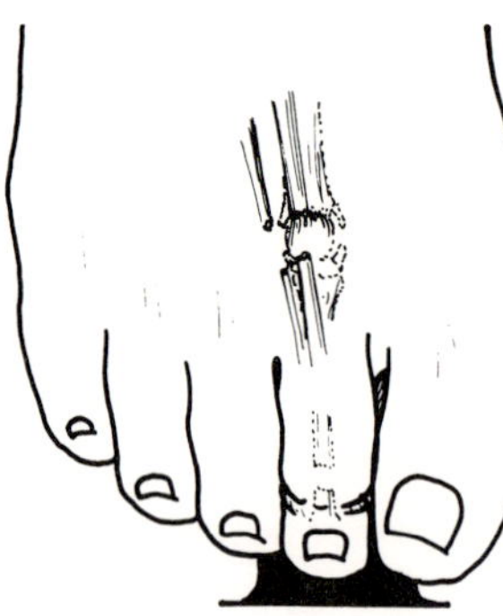

FIGURE 4

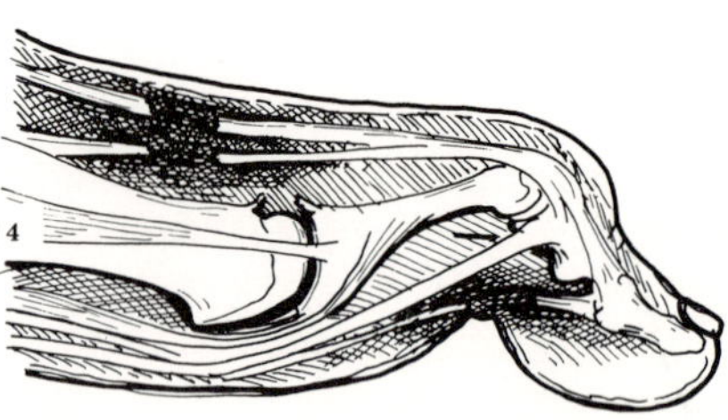

continued dorsal elevation of the tenotome, the paired short flexor tendons can be pinned against the joint and cut (Fig. 5). The digit will be straightened by long and short tenotomy

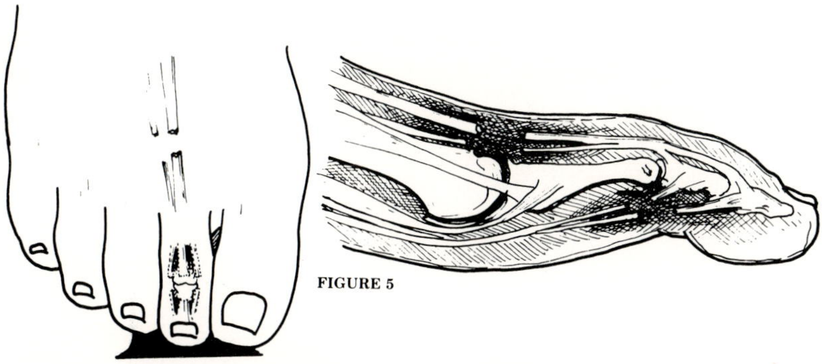

FIGURE 5

except for renmant flexion contracture of the capsule and this is eliminated by further, firm capsulotomy while the joint is forcibly extended by the surgeon. (Fig. 6).

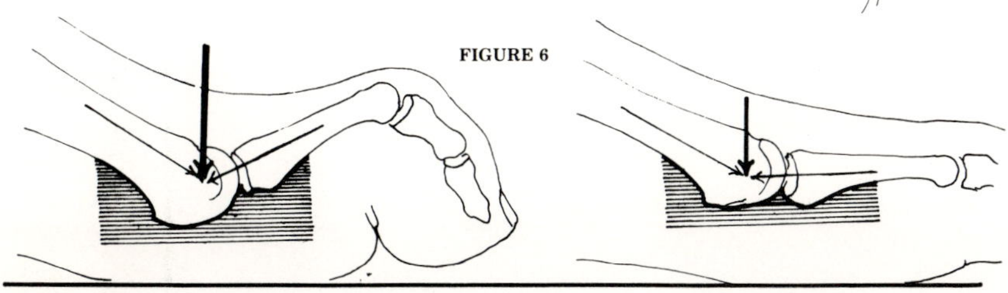

FIGURE 6

Postoperative Management

The simple surgical release of tendon and capsular tension must be followed by persistent retention of improved alignment to prevent future recurrence and heightened deformity. The urethane mold splint has provided a simple, optimal means of postoperative toe splinting but any similar device or technique which serves the purpose should be instituted. Depending on chronicity, realigned digits must be maintained for several months to a year. The importance of posture and optimal foot balance in rehabilitation of the forefoot has already been indicated. Functional guides, tarsal stablizers, and accommodative orthotics are provided to serve this purpose.

Proper shoes should be prescribed and insisted upon as a vital part of the restorative program.

Advantage

1. Soft tissue release represents a fully ambulatory procedure, without disability.

SECTION V

PROCEDURES LESS COMMONLY PERFORMED FOR IPK

A. Peg and Hole Procedure

In reviewing the literature one is amazed at the wide variety of surgical procedures for correction of an intractable plantar keratoma which are no longer in vogue. Dissatisfaction with the procedure for any number of reasons has caused these procedures to be discarded. One such surgical procedure was known as the "peg-in-hole". The following is a brief description of the procedure and a critique of why it is no longer considered a good procedure.

Surgical Procedure

The peg-in-hole technique for shortening of a lesser metatarsal for correction of an intractable plantar keratoma was first recommended by D. McKeever in 1952. The technique consisted of a dorsal linear incision centered over the metatarsal neck exposing the metatarso-phalangeal joint and the distal aspect of the metatarsal shaft. The metatarsal is divided, with a saw, transversly through its neck. Beginning on its raw surface a drill hole in the metatarsal head is made ¼ inch in diamenter and deep enough to allow the desired amount of shortening for the metatarsal. Then the distal end of the metatarsal shaft is rounded and firmly impacted into the hole in the head. The two fragments must fit together snugly or they may become separated later. Should the fixation seem insecure internal or external fixation could be employed. Some form of cast immobilization is used postoperatively.

Advantages

The literature relates that this procedure has certain advantages; however, their comparison was to resection of the metatarsal head which has been shown to have disasterous effects postoperatively.

1. Preserves the metatarsal head
2. Preserves the metatarso-phalangeal joint
3. Usually requires no form of fixation
4. Shortens a long metatarsal

Disadvantages

1. Limitation of motion of the involved metatarso-phalangeal joint postoperatively.
2. Loss of weight bearing function of metatarsal at times.
3. Occurence of transfer lesions to adjacent metatarsal head areas if metatarsal is shortened too much.
4. Shortens the metatarsal, which could prove disasterous in a normal or already shortened metatarsal.
5. Possible psuedoarthrosis due to improper remodeling and fixation of fragment.
6. Difficulty of performing surgery.
7. Need bone of good density.
8. Prolonged disability with immobilization.

Bibliography

McKeever, D. C.: Arthrodesis of the first metatarso-phalangeal joint for hallux valgus, hallux rigidus, and metatarsus primus varus. *J. Bone Joint Surg.*, **34A**:129, 1952.

Campbell: *Operative Orthopedics*, 5th ed. (A. H. Crenshaw, Editor) C. V. Mosby Co., St. Louis, 1971, pp. 1832-1834.

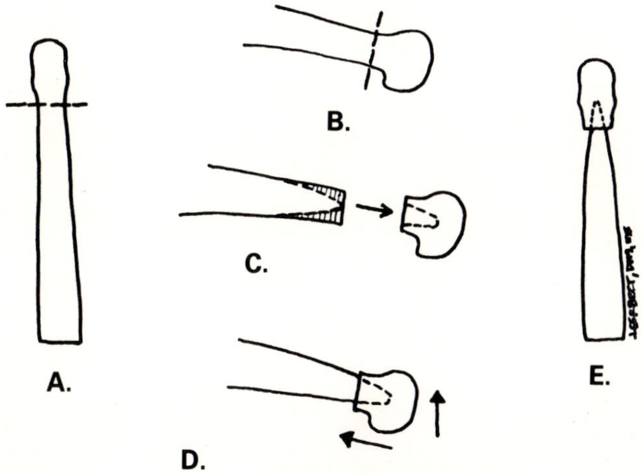

FIGURE 1
PEG AND HOLE PROCEDURE

This diagram demonstrates the primary steps in performing a peg and hole procedure for elimination of an intractable plantar keratoma.

A. This is a dorsal view of a lesser metatarsal showing the approximate area through the metatarsal neck that the osteotomy is made.

B. This is a lateral view of the area in which the osteotomy is made.

C. This diagram shows how one remodels the metatarsal shaft into a cone-shaped configuration and a compliment drill hole is made into the metatarsal head.

D. This demonstrates the two fragments united and that one achieves shortening as well as dorsiflexion.

E. This is a dorsal view showing the two fragments united.

B. Floating of the Metatarsals

Preoperative Signs

1. Fibrous or nucleated fibrous shearing callous.
2. Plantarly prominent metatarsal head.

Preoperative Symptoms

1. A plantar hyperkeratotic lesion located under one or more metatarsal head areas, which has not responded to conservative treatment.
2. Pain in the hyperkeratotic lesion.
3. Burning or paraesthesias in the plantar lesion.
4. Swelling around the plantar lesion.
5. Thick plantar skin which the patient objects to.

Biomechanical Evaluation

1. Forefoot varus with hypermobile first ray.
2. Plantarly prominent metatarsal head.
3. This procedure can be performed only in cases where orthotic control can be instituted.

Preoperative X-ray Evaluation

1. Structurally sound metatarso-phalangeal joint.
2. May be excessively long metatarsal.
3. May be adjacent to excessively short metatarsal.

Surgical Procedure

The surgical procedure employed is basically identical to that used in dorsal closing wedge osteotomy. The main differences lie in angulation of the cut and the absence of fixation in a "floating" procedure. The skin incision is made at the area of the proximal portion of the metatarsal shaft. The subcutaneous tissue is dissected to the level of the proximal shaft. Here, the shaft is transected completely from dorsal to plantar. There is no attempt at fixation, and the only caution to make is that the osteotomy be performed at a 15° Dorso-Plantar angle to prevent postoperative dislocation.

Postoperative Management

Postoperative management basically involves a dressing correction to maintain the corrected position. The dressing employed can be of felt, or plaster. The correction must be maintained for a period of 4-6 weeks in order to allow for healing in the corrected position.

Advantages

1. Metatarsal seeks its own level.
2. No wedge is removed thereby preserving length.

Disadvantages

1. Inability to maintain proper position.
2. Postoperative lesion transfere due to a too high or too low position.

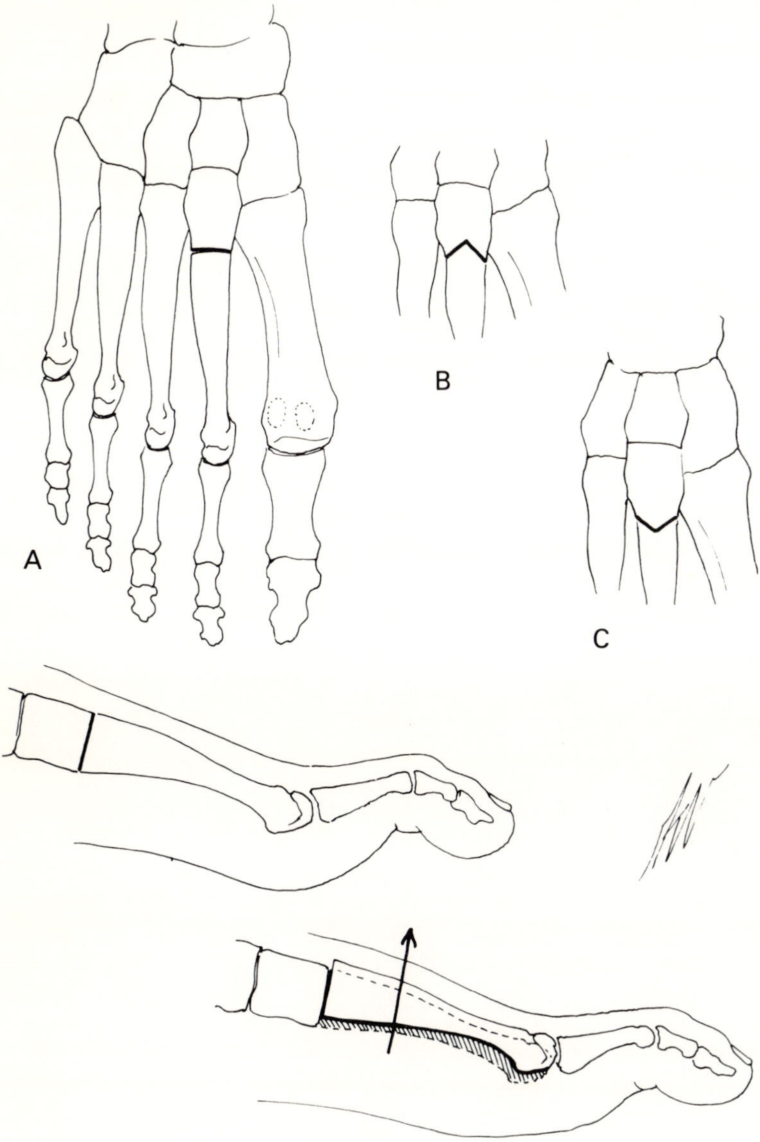

FIGURE 1

This figure represents two varieties of floating of the metatarsals. A) represents a linear cut at the base in an effort to release the metatarsal; C) and B) represent "V" shaped osteotomies at the base. The purpose of either technique is to allow the metatarsal to seek its own level with no fixation.

C. Metatarsal Collectomy

This procedure is a "gap ostectomy" at the anatomic neck region of a lesser metatarsal bone for the resolution of an established, intractable plantar lesion. It was devised by Dr. Alan Whitney in 1963 and no previous reference to a similar technique has been reported. The selective resection of a lesser metatarsal neck represents an intentional non-union to relieve excessive pressure upon the chronic plantar lesion.

Preoperative Symptoms

1. Pain occurs on weightbearing, with or without shoes.
2. Lateral digital compression induces sharp pain.

Biomechanical Evaluation

1. Excessive metatarsal length or relative protrusion.
2. Metatarsal declination deviation from nornal.
3. Metatarsus adductus, latus, and torsional abnormality.

Preoperative X-ray Evaluation

1. Metatarsal length pattern aberration.
2. Hyperdeclination of the involved segment.
3. Metatarsus adductus angle and individual splay angles.

Surgical Procedure

A dorsal longitudinal skin incision of 3 cm. length is made centrally over the anatomic neck of the selected metatarsal bone. A second fascial incision is performed to reach the level of the extensor tendon sheath which is incised to permit retraction of the long tendon under the medial or lateral skin margin. The metatarsal neck, now in view, is bluntly denuded of its fibroperiosteal sheath with a small periosteal elevator. With strong bone-cutting forceps or a rotary bone saw, the proximal transverse neck division is performed at a level 1 cm. proximal of the discernible head-neck junction. The distal divided fragment can then be elevated for the second transverse division at the head-neck junction level, with your bone-cutting instruments. The isolated neck section, of approximately 1 cm. length, is extracted and the remaining bone ends inspected and smoothed as necessary. Subcutaneous fascial closure is attained by three or four plain catgut (000) sutures. Several simple interrupted silk (000) sutures serve for skin approximation. A sponge dressing, overlaid with circular bandage under moderate tension is applied.

Postoperative Management

Redressing is performed in three days. The patient can return to a moderate occupation almost immediately. The sutures may be removed in ten days. Orthotics should be applied within the first postoperative month for the control of foot malalignment and imbalance.

Advantages

1. A fully ambulatory procedure that is suitable for office surgery or outpatient facilities.
2. Avoidance of intra-articular intervention.
3. Requires no fixation or splinting.

Disadvantages

1. Presumably unsuited for the first metatarsal segment.
2. Is not reconstructive in the sense of realignment by fixation-osteotomy where such is possible or essential.
3. Does not correct or improve associated metatarso-phalangeal subluxation or dislocation.
4. Transfer lesions possible.
5. Shortening of involved digit.
6. Does not correct a dorsiflexed MP joint that is ankylosed.
7. A painful MP joint preoperatively may persist postoperatively.

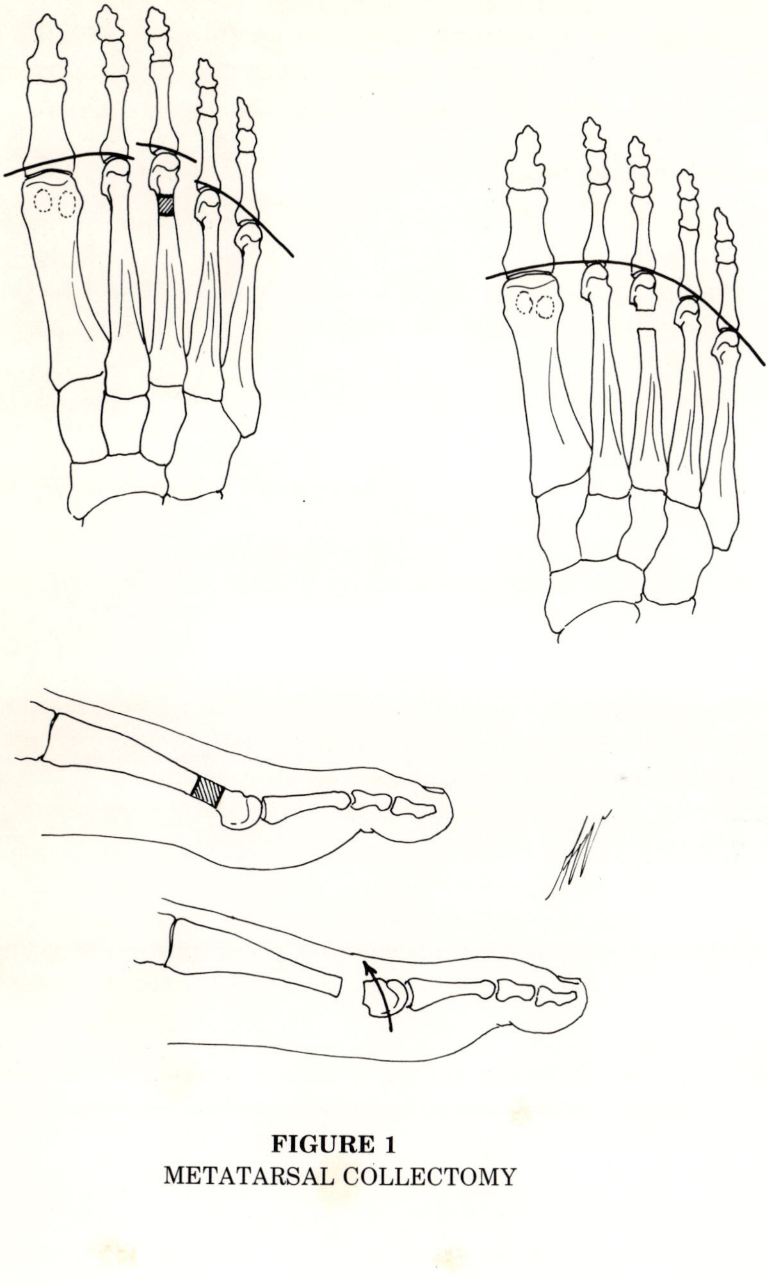

FIGURE 1
METATARSAL COLLECTOMY